One Step Ahead

Of Parkinson's Disease

Matt Wilbur

ISBN-131477646493 / 9781477646496

Front cover: Matt Wilbur, Kristen Martin and Mike Dubin
                 2011 New York City Marathon

Pictures on front and back cover provided by Kristen Martin

Scripture verses taken from The NIV Study Bible
                 Copyright 1985
                 By The Zondervan Corporation

The 1977 edition of *The Book of Lists* by David Wallechinsky, Irving Wallace and
                 Amy Wallace pp. 469-470

This book is dedicated to
Julie, Kristen, and Cory

Table of Contents

Preface

I am just an average kind of a guy. I am not a professional, Olympic or collegiate athlete. I am a retired high school math teacher and coach, who has been a recreational runner for thirty-five years. I am just like the guy you see running down your street when you look out your living room window. The only difference is that I am probably a little older, a lot slower, and I have Parkinson's disease.

I began running back in the 1970s. I became a pretty good marathon runner with a PR (Personal Record) of 2:59:40. My life changed in 2002, when I was diagnosed with Parkinson's disease.

In 2009, I decided to run the New York City Marathon for the Michael J. Fox Foundation for Parkinson's Research. I found that there was not a lot of information written about people who run marathons with Parkinson's. There just were not a lot of us out there.

After running the New York City Marathon for Team Fox, I started to speak to others about my journey. I started to think that there might be people out there that felt like I did. Maybe others might want to do something like running a marathon… something that would affirm that Parkinson's may have slowed them down; they are still "One Step Ahead." This was the motivation for my writing of this book.

None of this could have been possible without the support of my wife Julie and my daughters, Kristen and Cory.

Part of the proceeds from the sale of this book will be donated to the Michael J. Fox Foundation for Parkinson's Research.

Growing Up Without Running

I grew up in an upper middle class community of Wyoming, Ohio (a suburb of Cincinnati). Wyoming is a town of about 8,500 people who reside on less than three square miles of residential real estate. Most of the people would be considered affluent and well educated. Wyoming prides itself in its residential beauty and its city schools. Wyoming High School is often rated on a list of "Top 100 Schools" in the nation. There are high standards. Students are expected to take a demanding college prep curriculum and to go off to a prestigious college or university. Growing up, I never heard the terms "career center" or "vocational education."

I mention this because it is only by chance that when my parents moved to Cincinnati in the early 1950s, they built a small house on the edge of town, never knowing the type of community they had chosen to raise their family. I also want to say that I never felt that I was good enough to meet the standards set by the community. Our house was nice, but modest compared to my peers. We bought our clothes from a Sears catalog instead of from a department store at the local mall. As a first born child, I always wanted to achieve. I took advanced classes in high school, but performed near the bottom of the class. I sat in the back row and tried not to make eye contact with the teacher in fear of being called upon. My College Board scores, although not bad for most students, did not measure up to most of my classmates. I felt embarrassed.

Athletically, Wyoming offered many opportunities to develop my future skills. My parents provided me with the chance to participate in Little League and YMCA basketball. They were a little afraid of youth football. My dad had little, if any, athletic ability. He didn't teach me how to hit, throw, catch or shoot. What I learned, I learned in the back yard with neighborhood friends or at the basketball hoop that was put up between two trees next to our driveway. I played on the better teams, but was never one of the better players. I was just good enough to be part of the team.

In high school, I played varsity football and basketball. In basketball, after playing on the 7th and 8th grade teams, I was cut during my freshman year. I came back out my sophomore season and made the team. When I was a senior, there were only three seniors on the team. Once again, I was good enough to be on the team, but that was it.

I never thought about running in high school. I knew that it was the football and basketball players who were popular and were all looked up to. I never understood why a student would want to run all those miles in cross country. Besides, during my senior year, I weighed about 190 lbs., which didn't give me the proper body type one needs to be a runner. I thought it was more fun drinking milkshakes from United Dairy Farmers trying to gain weight for football.

My athletic experience, although not glorious, still had a huge impact on my future professional career choice. I decided to teach high school mathematics and to become a coach. Once again, although an honorable profession, I was embarrassed to tell my classmates who were going into professions such as medicine, law, or politics. (At least, that is the way I perceived it.)

After graduating from Wyoming High School in 1971, I attended Miami University in Oxford, Ohio. I was scared to death that I wouldn't be prepared. I also felt that since I was paying a lot of money for this education, I had the responsibility to get my money's worth and to be successful. I was pretty serious about my studies and did not do a lot of the typical college social stuff. I just hung out with a few of my friends. I quickly realized how well Wyoming had prepared me, as my grades were consistently A's and B's. I was on the Dean's List along with the President's List of Distinguished Scholars several times, and graduated Cum Laude with a 3.5 GPA. That was one thing I was proud of and felt I earned.

I also spent about a year and a half as part of NROTC (Naval Reserve Officer Training Corps). I walked into their offices the first week of school to see about getting into the program so that the government couldn't take my low draft number and give me a ticket to the Viet Nam War. The military was never a topic for discussion at any point while I was growing up. The Navy not only accepted me, it also gave me a scholarship which added to my commitment. It paid my tuition, books and $100 a month stipend. I was surprised that between my academic success and my unrealized leadership skills, they believed that I was good officer material. Something about the discipline appealed to me. Some of my first experiences with running came during the physical training involved in the program. I actually went on NATO maneuvers in Norway the summer after my freshman year. I couldn't get used to grown men saluting me and saying, "Sir". I could not see myself fitting into a military career. When the Viet Nam War was over, and it was permissible to withdraw without any penalty, I decided to do so and regained a "normal civilian" status.

When I graduated from Miami University in 1975 with a degree in mathematics education and a minor in physical education, I felt that I was ready to conquer the world of education and the coaching profession. I accepted a teaching job in Mount Vernon, Ohio. I was going to be a high school math teacher and a varsity assistant football coach. I was also fortunate to be hired as a men's assistant basketball coach at Kenyon College in Gambier, Ohio, which was right outside of Mount Vernon. I thought I was ready to take on the world. Bring it on.

After one year on my own, I decided to ask a young woman I had dated at Miami University, Julie Deevers, to marry me. We met in an anatomy class, which was a physical education requirement. I was a "front row" student and she and her friend were in the back row, usually giggling. As we got to know each other, I realized how similar our values and goals were. We dated for a couple of years. It was probably selfish not to discuss marriage during college and possibly getting married right after graduation, but I wanted to have a year by myself and see what else there was in the world. I was very fortunate that she said "yes."

Married life must have agreed with me, because within a year, my weight had climbed to about 205 lbs. and was rising. My clothes must have started to shrink when Julie washed them because they started to get tight on me. The thought of running to reduce weight had begun to enter my mind. On New Year's Eve, 1977, I decided I would try this thing they called "jogging". It didn't begin on January 2nd, but it was now a goal that would soon become a reality and would be part of my life for the next thirty-five years. I never could have imagined the journey that running would take me on or the impact it would have on my life.

Becoming a runner is by nature, a selfish pursuit. It is basically an individual choice that requires many hours away from your spouse and family. Weekends often require large blocks of time, not just the hours to run, but the time to prepare, often travel time to meet with others with whom you plan to spend "quality" time. And then of course, the time required to recover, lying around the house most of the day. Times you travel (to your in-laws for instance) may cause stress because they won't understand the reason you are so impolite as to change into your running clothes and go out for a "much needed" run instead of visiting with family members. These actions, although seen as necessary by you, are not understood by others and can very easily cause stress between your spouse and family. If you as a runner are honest with yourself, there are probably times when you are trying to "run" away from the responsibilities you face as a member of this social institution we call a family. I don't have all the answers to this social dilemma, but priorities must be determined by everyone involved. Compromises and being flexible with your time will go a long way toward relieving the tension.

Learning on the Run

I would guess that by March, 1978, I was ready to get started to become a runner, but I wondered where do I start. The culture of runners was almost nonexistent. Those people one did see running were considered weird or different to say the least.

I remember my first run in the spring of 1978. I had already taken my car and found that the fire hydrant down the street was one half mile from our house. I found an old pair of gym shorts from college, a white t-shirt, a pair of tube socks with colored stripes around the top, laced up my Chuck Taylor All-Star basketball shoes that I coached in at Kenyon, and ran to the fire hydrant and back. That was my first mile. That wasn't bad.

Clothing and Apparel

There was not much of a market for running shoes and apparel. I remember the time I went to the local sporting goods dealer and checked out his limited supply of running shoes. My first pair of shoes was a pair of Nike Cortez. They probably were not that great of a shoe for me (I remember them being a little snug in the toes), but I went home feeling like I was going to the Olympics. They had white leather uppers with that red Nike swoosh. They were so cool. Just as a side note… these are the same shoes worn by Forrest as he ran back and forth across America in the movie *Forrest Gump*.

I remember my first winter of running. I wore tube socks, a flannel undershirt, sweat pants, maybe a sweatshirt, followed by the oldest winter coat that I could find in my closet. This ensemble was complemented with a scarf, a ski mask, and a pair of socks to cover my hands.

I used to reward myself for meeting certain running goals (running for a month for example) by allowing myself to purchase some type of running gear. I was not sure how long I was going to stay with this running life, so investing in apparel made it easier to keep running. Maybe I would buy an actual pair of running socks, some nylon running shorts with a slit up the side that made one look real sexy, or a running singlet that made me look like a real runner at races. I was like most new runners. When I went to a race, I pinned my race number on a t-shirt, probably on the back. At one point, I bought a singlet that had a meshed middle that enabled me to cool off in the summer. I considered it "state-of-the art" clothing.

Over the years there has been a huge growth in the market for running clothes that uses the latest technology to improve performance. Materials changed and improved the ability to wick sweat away from the body, therefore having the desired cooling effect. I remember the first time I wore running tights; I was so self-conscious that I wore a pair of shorts over the top of the tights. Running outfits now can keep you cooler in the summer and warmer in the winter with much more comfort than in earlier days. There are now dozens of shoe companies competing in the running market. Shoes are made to meet the many needs of runners: training, racing, track, trail running, and cross training. They are also made to match one's particular biomechanical needs: stability, performance, neutral, or motion control shoes are made by almost every company.

Electronics has also had an impact on the running community. Music has always served a purpose in athletic training. It can be a great motivational tool. The means for listening to this music while running has changed over the years, from the Walkman to MP3 players and the IPod, all of which have made listening to music a simple task. I have used all of these music devices in the past, but recently I decided I wanted to enjoy the total sensual experience running provides. Many fitness centers have televisions to watch while one runs on a treadmill. Runners are able to wear a heart monitor to study the proper heart rate at which to train. A simple watch was replaced by a chronograph which included many functions that could measure different information such as: time of day, running time, a timer that rings at pre-set intervals, and an alarm clock. You need to be a computer geek to understand it all. Runners can now wear a GPS type watch that measures such things as: elapsed time, distance run, instantaneous pace, overall pace and pulse. All this information can then be downloaded onto a computer to analyze.

Learning

On the world stage of running in the 1970s, Americans were the lead dogs. Runners like Bill Rogers (a 4 time winner of the Boston and New York City Marathons during the 1970s); Frank Shorter (won a gold medal at the 1972 Olympic marathon and a silver medal at the 1976 Olympic marathon); Steve Prefontaine and Marty Lequori (American middle distance runners), all became running cult heroes. These were young men that we novice runners began to read about and maybe see run on Wide World of Sports with Jim McKay. There were no sports channels such as ESPN.

Those of us who began running in the late 1970s had to learn to run on the fly. I started to read popular running books of the day. *The*

5

Complete Book of Running by James Fixx was the first book I read that was a great resource for beginning runners. It had a red cover with a pair of running legs on the front, which really made it stand out. When Fixx died of a heart attack, this provided evidence for those who didn't want to buy into this running lifestyle.

Jeff Galloway wrote a book *Galloway's Book on Running* which was the first book that I read that laid out a plan for walkers or joggers and told them what they needed to do over about a thirty week program to run the marathon. He even laid out plans for those who wanted to run it in a particular time. Reading this book sparked an interest in me to run a marathon. What an accomplishment that would be! Was it possible that a normal, recreational runner could run a marathon?

Dr. George Sheehan wrote several books, the best of which I felt was *Running and Being, The Total Experience*. Sheehan was not only a runner; he was a philosopher of sorts. He was like a guru to some of us in the running community. He investigated the right side of the runner's brain. He explored the beauty and peace found by running and stated that each of us was meant to be an athlete, not a spectator.

One of the best resources I used was from a monthly magazine that began publishing in the 1970s called *Runner's World*. It has been a source of information about all areas of running as well as providing inspirational and motivational material for me since that time.

There was also a lot of scientific research being done by Dr. Kenneth Cooper in Texas who was finding empirical evidence that supported the advantages of making exercise part of a personal lifestyle. He was trying to prove what all runners already knew. Cooper was credited with introducing the term "aerobics" into our culture.

Training

I started running at a turning point in the history of athletics. "Baby Boomers" all over the country began to exercise for personal reasons: to lose weight (that was a big one), to relieve stress we were putting on ourselves, pursuing a lifestyle we thought would bring us happiness. Many wanted to add a new mental, almost spiritual dimension to their lives. Whatever the reason, we were all part of a new social phenomenon known as the "Running Boom". Runners could now be seen anywhere, at any time of the day or night and in any kind of weather.

When I read Jeff Galloway's book, I put together a plan, running by time not by miles. I might run 45 minutes on Monday, Wednesday, and Friday, 30 minutes on Tuesday and Thursday, and 60 minutes on Sunday. After several months, I realized that a 45 minute run would cover about 6 miles. I did this for most of 1978 and ran approximately

900 miles that first year. I kept track of my first year's running on notebook paper and I would thumb tack it to the wall next to the kitchen phone.

I never really ran what one would call a long run of more than 16 miles, but I did put in some large mileage weeks of over 50 miles. A basic training run might consist of an 8 mile run which I could easily complete in one hour. I also started to incorporate hill training and interval training on alternate weeks.

The term "cross training" became part of any training program. Runners found that if they ran hard every day, injuries were right around the corner. Not only were rest days important, but an alternative form of aerobic activity was sometimes added to one's workout schedule. Weight training, use of a treadmill, elliptical trainers (less impact but a good aerobic workout), biking, deep water running (I could never figure that one out) or low impact form running on a small trampoline were all experimented with. I found that weight training was beneficial at all times and I would use the others at various times, usually when rehabbing from an injury of some sort. I had a habit of using some of these when I got tired of running, thinking that it was of equal in benefit. I found that if I wanted to become a good runner, I had to run, period. The others are good add-ons, but they cannot replace running.

Running had really taken a hold of me and was changing my life in a lot of ways. It was almost like a religious conversion experience. By January 1, 1979, I was keeping a runner's log, recording all of the pertinent information about my running experience. My wife made it a habit to give me a new one each Christmas. I was taking my running lifestyle very seriously. In my first year of running, my weight went from 205 lbs. to 167 lbs. My coaching buddies called me "bird cage" because my ribs showed through my skin. I started to investigate my nutritional needs. I started to make my own yogurt and granola. I experimented with fasting one day a week. I also tried carbohydrate loading, including the depletion stage, which was pretty tough on the body. I took it as a compliment when people said I looked sickly, because that is the way all good runners seemed to look.

I was not a real creative, free-thinking, run-as-you feel kind of a runner. I had certain routes that I ran almost all of the time based on what was called for on a particular day. If I wanted to go:

2 miles: YMCA and home
3 miles: Viaduct and home
4 miles: Burger King and home
5 miles: High School and home
6 miles: Mount Vernon Nazarene University and home
7 miles: Same as 6 miles + neighborhood

8   miles: Riverside Park to high school to Gay St. and home
9   miles: Riverside Park to high school to shopping center and home
10 miles: Same as 9 miles but Sanitarian Rd. and home

On all of these runs, I needed to have a plan for taking care of bodily functions. I needed to know where I could get a drink. Water was at Riverside Park, Beck's Drive-In, Wendy's, Memorial Park, the swimming pool and Dan Emmett School. I also needed to know where I could find a restroom. They were available at Riverside and Memorial Parks, local gas stations, fast food places, the high school and at the swimming pool during open hours. There were times when I was not near a convenient place and I just had to use whatever Mother Nature had to offer. I'd jump behind a local tree or bush and hope nobody would see me and that there would be some wide leaves available that were not poison ivy. Social etiquette is a little different while I run in regards to spitting and blowing my nose. There were many times well intentioned people would call Julie and tell her they had just seen me throwing up somewhere. Stuff happens!

I was very fortunate, while living in Mount Vernon, to have access to a beautiful bike path. The Kokosing Gap Trail was built on an old train rail bed. It was about 15 miles long and went through the woods along the Kokosing River, through the outdoor athletics facilities at Kenyon College and then through some of Knox County's rural countryside, ending near Danville.

The trail was marked each ½ mile and was as flat as anyone would want. It also had water and restrooms near the start and at Kenyon College which was at the 4 ½ mile mark. The beginning of the trail was 2 ½ miles from my house, so on longer runs I would run from my house to the bike path, go a certain distance on the path, turn around and come home. It also meant that if I wanted to increase my long run by 2 miles, it meant I only had to go one more mile out on the bike path and then home. It would give me a psychological lift. It worked for me.

Maybe it just worked out this way, but unless a person has a plan to run more than one marathon in a year, it is best to cycle one's training. Having a build-up period of approximately three months, a period of five to six months of high mileage and strength training, running the marathon, and then taking about three months to recover is doable in the long run. It is hard to start over each year, but training hard without change and rest for more than a year will eventually lead to injuries.

Running Groups

I started to find a few other guys like me who were also starting to run. Terry Bush, whose family was like having a family in Mount

Vernon, also began to run about that same time. We ran a lot together. When we ran, very rarely was it in an organized way. We didn't know where we were going to go until we talked about how far we needed to go depending on how our training was going. On those runs we would share what we had learned. We'd talk about our goals, races that were coming up or about getting faster. If we found ourselves not talking, it probably meant we were running too fast. We'd find ourselves running races together. Races like The Mavis 5 Mile Run in Mount Vernon, as well as other races in the area, always offered a new challenge. We always compared times and there was always a friendly competition among all of us. Guys like Terry Bush, Nick Frost, Bill Ernst, Don Muncie, and Tom Nagy not only competed against each other, but also shared information that would make us better. And we got better. Running groups are great unless someone is mad at one of the other runners and turns it into an "I'll show you" kind of a run, and then picks up the pace to a level where one doesn't want to go. This has happened a few times and the best thing I found to do was to let them take off, let them prove their point, and then pick it up together the next time. I learned that I don't ever want to cut a runner out of my life; they may be able to help somewhere in the future.

Setting Goals

I found myself setting goals at the start of each year and writing them on the first page of a new year's runner's log. Goals gave me something to strive for, to dream about, to visualize, and to enjoy when they were accomplished. I had some goals that were easy to accomplish, some were average in difficulty, and some where things were going to have to go just right for them to be accomplished. That way there was almost always something to feel good about each year. Over a period of several years, I found that when I didn't write down my goals, things usually didn't go as well that year.

There are a few other areas of running that need to be mentioned before we look at the highlights (and low points) of my running career.

Injuries and Other Ouchies

Injuries are going to happen. Injuries are just accidents in the big scheme of things, but sometimes we can do things in a proactive way in order to give ourselves the best chance to avoid injuries. Stretching was a positive when I was running at a high level, especially in terms of speed. Slow static stretching was valuable. I stretched before I ran as a transition from my hectic life to my time of running. It is probably beneficial to stretch after a run, but time and sweating on the living room carpet sometimes eliminates that as an option.

During the past few years, the Galloway Training Program has discouraged stretching. Jeff Galloway said that there was no evidence that stretching was beneficial and that in fact, it may be harmful. The speed at which I trained in 2012, during the first 20 minutes or so of running seemed to loosen up the muscles adequately.

One should always be careful when increasing either mileage or the speed at which you train. If we are trying to go farther or faster, it shows that we are motivated, but sometimes we don't use good discretion. If we miss a workout it is usually not a good idea to just jump ahead. Once it's gone, let it go, and just continue with the program. When I put a plan together, I usually give myself a few extra weeks in case unforeseen setbacks occur.

Getting the proper nutrition and rest, although difficult to do, is very helpful. One would think that it would be a no-brainer, but it took a while to realize that I could run well when I took my medications as prescribed for the day, instead of skipping some of the doses. Imagine that. It seems that we have a tendency to add stress onto stress and eventually something has to give.

It seems that whenever I am on the cusp of a terrific athletic accomplishment, when I am in the best of conditioning, that's when I am most susceptible to injuries. I have had my share of injuries. The difficulty is deciding whether what I am exhibiting is just an "ouchie" that I can probably run through, or if it is an injury and I need to rest in order to avoid further damage. I have experienced a lot of common physical setbacks:

1) Blood blisters
2) Chaffed nipples, crotch, and underarms
3) Blackened toenails (one must get the blood out and watch it fall off)
4) Bruised heel (very painful)
5) Sprained ankle
6) Strained ligaments around the knee
7) Overall fatigue from inadequate recovery
8) Stress fracture (required weeks on crutches)

When a pain develops, that is a good time to think about either buying a new pair of shoes, or whether I have been overtraining. Anti-inflammatory medicines like Tylenol, Aleve, and Advil are all standard issue for any runner, as well as a freezer full of ice.

Weight Control

Maybe it's just the mathematician in me, but I always felt that weight can tell you a lot. From a physics standpoint, it seems logical that the less weight one has to carry, the easier the running would become. I found that when I run consistently, the weight will come off. When I run, I burn about 100 calories per mile, so if I run a 30 mile week, I can lose about a pound. It takes burning about 3,000 - 3,500 calories to lose a pound.

Looking at one's weight over time gives an indication of how one's training is going. As we age, our metabolism slows down, so although running speeds up the metabolism, I found that dieting probably is needed to lose weight. I have tried several diets: The Zone Diet, The Slim Fast Plan, and the "Just Eat Less" diet. I have found that the Slim Fast Plan, with two drinks and a couple of zone bars for snacks and a reasonable dinner worked well for me. I also found that when dieting, the body will slow down its metabolism because the brain thinks it's starving. Therefore, I alternate between diet days and normal days in hopes of confusing the body's reaction to starvation. A good guide is to try to weigh what one weighed in high school.

Vacations

Going on a family vacation while in the middle of a running program can be difficult. How do you fit running into the time with your family? Running is a selfish activity and your family deserves some time with you void of a running schedule. But what if you think that you can't take two weeks away from running? What do you do? If you stay in a hotel that has a fitness center with a treadmill, that's a possibility, but you should schedule it before everybody wakes up. I usually just cut back and pick it up when I get home. You are the one who needs to sacrifice. If you really want a successful vacation, give your family the time they deserve.

Galloway Training Program

Jeff Galloway gave me my first marathon training program back in the 1970s and I used it for many years. But his program has changed drastically. In 2011, after returning to Cincinnati, I began training with the Cincinnati Galloway Training Group. The new concepts seemed like it was designed for my needs. It incorporated running and walking together in a predetermined run/walk ratio. For example, good runners might run four minutes and walk a minute. Others might run two minutes and walk a minute. I found that running a minute and walking a minute worked well for me. I realized that I am walking half the marathon and if I want a fast time, I need to learn to walk fast.

The previous two years before joining Galloway Training Group, running was difficult because there was no one that ran as slowly as I did, therefore I'd have a lot of long runs by myself. With the Cincinnati Galloway Group, there was always someone willing to run with me. There was security in knowing that I would never be left behind. Many Saturday mornings, Larry Snowden and Bill Theis sacrificed their own time to make sure I got through our prescribed run.

Running Highlights

After thirty-five years of running, I have experienced many of life's highs and lows. I have learned there is another world outside of running. Only when I look at the total picture, do I realize how one impacts the other. Running has truly had a tremendous impact on my life. It has enriched my life. It has given me more strength to battle the physical demons I face every day. I am much healthier because of the cumulative effect of thirty-five years of running. Running is like a sieve. Running an hour after a day filled with the stresses of the world I think I want, I find that after sixty minutes of running, the bad stuff will be sifted away and what is left is worth keeping.

In the following pages, I will try to show you both of my worlds: the world of running and how it coexisted with my real world. I have written these highlights in outline format as they appeared in my runner's logs. It is important to understand that these entries are not intended in any way to be a guide to marathon training. This was a journey of one average recreational runner, what I learned along the way, and the impact it had on my life.

All of these experiences prepared me for the journey that I now find myself on. My life is better in 2012 because of the foundation that was laid in all those years of running. I am fortunate that I still have the strength and the will to run. I still have a desire to get faster and stronger every day, but my running has now taken on a whole new meaning in my life. I hope that my running life can have an impact on the lives of others, not just to run, but to live an excellent life that we were all created for. Enjoy the journey.

1979

Goals:

1)   Run three marathons in 1979
2)   Run a 5 mile race in 30 minutes
3)   Run 1500 miles
4)   Still be running in December

January 1:   Ran 5 miles with Terry Bush at 7:00 pm – good start

February 18:   ***5 Mile Race at Kenyon College Fieldhouse***

        16 guys ran - I finished 1st in 31:32, Nick was 2nd, Terry was 3rd

March 25:   Highest weekly mileage of 54 miles – weight is 163

April 1:   ***Athens Marathon in Athens, Ohio***

Well, this is it. Terry and I wondered what this would be like. We had no idea what we were in for. We had just read about running a marathon. There were probably a couple of hundred runners with very few women. We went out in about a 7 min./mile pace and it felt very easy. I remember running on a country road with people sitting in their front yards with hoses offering us water. It was basically an out and back course, and I kept asking myself, "Where is this thing they refer to as 'The Wall'?" At about mile 17, I thought it might be a good idea to stop and stretch a bit. That idea stayed constant throughout the rest of the race. Pretty soon I was convinced that walking a little and then running a little was a good idea. I had been introduced to the "Survival Shuffle". It would be a constant companion in future marathons. I later realized that these physiological changes and adaptations were what are referred to as "Hitting the Wall". I was happy to finally enter Ohio University football stadium feeling like I was entering the Olympic stadium. I finished in 3:24. Terry finished in 3:31. It was a great experience.

May 5:   ***Kristen Michelle Wilbur*** *entered the world during the Kentucky Derby. This was one of the most significant days of my life. Could I be the kind of a father she needed? As a teacher I saw hundreds of kids each year. I observed the "good" kids that I saw in school and tried to find the common denominators that made them turn out the way they did. I found that there are no absolutes, but I was going to play the odds. It seemed that the ones with a solid set of parents, where commitment was a reality, raising the children in a church, and having them know that the church was a vital part of our lives, was where I was going to invest my efforts. I have been happy with the return on the investment.*

Kristen has become a wonderful lady and mother. She is better than I ever deserved.

She was not much of an athlete in high school. She went out for track as a senior because her boyfriend was on the team. She was assigned to the distance runners and waved to the crowd from the back of the pack. It wasn't a total waste of time though. She married that high school boyfriend and they have a wonderful family.

She would become a marathoner after she was married like her dad and would play a major role in my running life in the years to come.

May 20:   Best week to date – 64 miles – 162 lbs.

June 3:   Ran twice a day this week – 73 miles (best week ever)

June 17: ***Glass City Marathon in Toledo, Ohio***

I finished in 3:18:48 which wasn't bad for 85 degree weather. I remember entering a stadium once again, but this time on the back straight away of the last lap, I threw up. Throwing up at the end of a race became a signature for me.

July 4:   ***Granville Firecracker 5 Mile Race***
98th out of 650 – 30:18

July 9:   Interval training: 10 x 440s @ 1:25; 5 x 220s @ :35 - :40

August 4:   ***Mavis 5 Mile Run*** - 30:14 (disappointing)

October 28:   ***Monroe Marathon***

Worst organized marathon I ever ran – course was out and back and then out and back again – not well attended- 37th out of 137 runners (3:22:04)

November 20:   Ran 5 miles in Kenyon College Fieldhouse after practice – last mile in 5:47

December 31:   Happy New Year – Ran 10 miles

Evaluation:

Not a bad year: 3 marathons – 1915 miles for the year

1980

Goals:

1) Run four marathons
2) Run a 3:10 marathon
3) Run a 5 Mile Race in 30 minutes
4) Run 2000 miles
5) Be running in December

February 17:   Best week of the year – 50 miles

March 16:   Ran 61 miles two weeks before Athens Marathon

March 23:   Ran 56 miles one week before Athens Marathon – not much of a taper

March 30:   ***Athens Marathon in Athens, Ohio***

Well-paced at 7:30/mile – plenty left in the tank at the end – finished 95/305 runners in a time of 3:21:02 – Terry struggled in 3:48

I started to think about these marathons I was investing in. One thought was that it appeared that I was consistently in about the top 25% - 30% of all runners. I never thought that a guy like me, who never ran before, could have that kind of success. Another thought was that there were so few women running the marathon. I realized that I usually could run with the best women runners. Things would change dramatically in terms of the number of and the talent level of women runners in the future.

May 18:   Ran 50 miles with five 8 mile runs – that is how I added mileage vs. running a longer run

I think that I was afraid of running a long run in training. I was very comfortable running 8 – 10 miles because I could do that in 1 hour – 1 hour 30 minutes and never leave town and always be close to home. If I wanted to go longer distances, it meant that I had to venture further from home and wrap my mind around the time commitment. I didn't want to go there.

May:	Had four consecutive weeks of: 50, 55, 62, and 59 miles – for me that is high mileage

June 15:	***Glass City Marathon in Toledo, Ohio***
	Ran a very good marathon – set a Personal Record (PR) of 3:11 – pretty good – Terry ran in 3:20

November 9:	Ran 65 miles for the week with a long run of 15 miles - short taper – last three days with no running

November 16:	***Columbus Bank One Marathon*** ***A Day to Remember – 2:59:40***

I found myself at the half-marathon mark having run several miles in 6:30 mins. /mile pace, and was looking at a time of 1:25. I had a major decision to make. I was five minutes ahead of a 3:00 marathon (one of the goals for a recreational runner). I had to decide whether to just finish, in what would surely be a PR, or do I go for it. I decided to go for it, as long as I could hold the necessary pace of 6:52 per mile. Although tiring, I found myself with a half mile to go and I needed an 8:00 pace to finish in 3:00. I remember verbally shouting, "I can't do this." A response came from the crowd on the curb. "You can do it, Matt." Startled I looked to my left and saw Julie cheering me on. I crossed the finish line, pushed "stop" on my chronograph, bent over, threw up and then checked my time. It was 2:59:40! I had run a 3:00 marathon by less than 1 second/mile. I didn't know it at the time, but this was as good as it would ever get. One never knows!

Evaluation:

I didn't achieve all of my goals – that's why I set several – some I achieve and some I keep striving for. I ran my best ever marathon in 2:59:40 (about a 6:52 mins. /mile). I ran 2018 miles (best year ever). My weight has started to inch up over 170 lbs. Should I get concerned? How good can I get? What are the limits to my running?

1981

Goals:

1)   Run 5 marathons
2)   Qualify for the Boston Marathon (requires a 2:50)
3)   Run 2200 miles
4)   Keep my weight in the 160 – 165 lbs. range
5)   Be running in December and enjoying it

Several things can slow down one's progress. One of those things is a personal change in your life outside of running that makes it difficult to train as you were accustomed. As much as we'd like to forget this, sometimes, we do have a life away from running that requires our attention. Different life stresses can alter our ability to improve.

In 1981, several of these things occurred in the same year. I had already cut back in the last two months of 1980 and had nagging injuries in the beginning of 1981. I also experienced a significant job change. I became the Head Boys' Basketball Coach at Loudonville High School. Although this was something I longed for professionally, the pressures and time required to do the job did cut into my training. I continued to live in Mount Vernon, so that meant an hour a day just driving.

A vicious cycle begins: I cut back my running, I begin to gain weight. My running becomes more difficult. It's harder to get the miles in because I'm carrying more weight, but I can't lose weight without increasing my mileage.

Jan.-March: Tried to deal with nagging injuries while increasing my long runs

April 5:   ***Athens Marathon in Athens, Ohio***

Disappointing – I finished in 3:27 – my heel is very sore my weight is 170 lbs. My heel will be sore for two more months (plantar fasciitis)

May 24:   ***Cleveland Revco 10K*** – finished in 41:15

June 21:   Heel is still sore

July 4:   **Granville Firecracker 5 Mile Run** – disappointing
                  31:18

August 15:   **Mavis 5 Mile Run**
                  hometown race – finished in 31:10

August: Very consistent month – ran 29/31 days – total 205
                  miles in August – weight down to 167 lbs. - If I run
                  consistently the weight will be under control.

October 11:   **Columbus Bank One Marathon**

                  I went out at a 6:30 mins. /mile pace and finished in
                  3:13:49 – still a respectable time.

Oct. – Dec.:   Didn't run another week over 20 miles

Evaluation:

> *The demands of my new coaching job as Head Basketball Coach have taken
> time away from the time I had for running. I ran 60 miles in November and
> 35 miles in December. My weight is up to 175 lbs. Things are not going
> well. You can't cheat the marathon. If you do the work, put in the miles,
> you have a chance that good things will happen, but if you don't do the work,
> it will eat you up and spit you out. I was still able to run 1700 miles and
> three marathons. Keep thinking positively.*

1982

Goals:

No written goals

When I can't run at a high level because of my job responsibilities, my mileage goes down, and my weight goes up. Maybe I'm just making excuses.

Evaluation:

Nothing of any significance happened other than minimal running – 867 miles – Am I in trouble?

1983

Goals:

No written goals

Jan. – March: Took three months to get to 100 miles of running – my weight is up to180 lbs.

April 24:   First 30 mile week

May 22:   First 40 mile week – triathlon training

May 23:   Graduated from Ashland College with a Master's degree in Education with a major in Sports Science

June: Ran 29/30 days

July 22:   ***Apple Valley Triathlon***

1000 meter swim in Apple Valley Lake - 20 miles on a bike around the lake - run 10K - finished in 2:23 (59th / 350) - very fun

October 10:   918 miles for the year

Oct. – Dec.:   Didn't run the rest of the year

Evaluation:

One triathlon - not much running – 918 miles – must get into a more demanding program

In 1982 I was scanning the television channels and ran across an athletic event that I had not seen before. It was called the "Ironman Triathlon." I couldn't believe what I saw these athletes doing. Each competitor had to swim 2.4 miles in the ocean, then get out of the water and ride a bike. They had to ride 115 miles and then run a marathon. Any one of the stages would have been enough. They had to complete the events before the cut off time of 17 hours.

As I watched, as millions of others did, a young woman named Julie Moss was leading the triathlon, well into the marathon. The announcers didn't really communicate what we were watching. Pretty soon we all saw Julie Moss start to fall apart. First she started to look like a deer that had been hit by a car. Staggering, she kept looking behind herself to see how much of a lead she had. Then one of the announcers stated, "She's starting to lose control of some of her bodily functions." Any endurance athlete who was watching saw her "poop" down her leg. As she approached the finish line, she became a total wreck. It was sad to watch. She collapsed a few yards from the finish line. The announcers were almost silent as she repeatedly tried to get up. Then in the blink of an eye, she was passed. She crawled to the finish line and finished in 2nd place.

The triathlon is really cool, but requires a lot of talent in three events and the resources to train and to compete in them effectively. It can be pretty expensive. I don't have any of the requirements to be successful in this endeavor.

1984

Goals:

No written goals

February 23:   First day of running of the year

Mar. – April: Started to run with the Loudonville Track Team – first 100 miles

May 19:   First 8 mile run

June: 165 miles for the month – ran 28/30 days (much better)

July 8:   Ran a 40 mile week – biked 65 miles – swam 4000 yards

August 11:   ***Mavis 5 Mile Run***

31:09 - not bad

August 19:   ***Apple Valley Triathlon***

Poor swim – good ride – average run

September 16:   Ran 14 miles – longest run in years

October 7:   ***Columbus Bank One Marathon***

Well-paced – finished in 3:08:35
No walks – where did that come from
Maybe good things can still happen

Nov. – Dec.:   Miles really came down drastically

Evaluation:

Not a bad year – worked hard and ran 1258 miles – good cross training - good marathon

1985

Goals:

No written goals

Jan. – March:	Total of 100 miles running
April:	116 miles for the month
June 10:	First 10 mile run – 43 mile week
June 30:	***Cory Deevers Wilbur is born in Bedford, Ohio***

Life is not fair. I hear it all the time. I didn't deserve this thing that has happened to me. Why did this thing happen to me?

That's exactly how I feel about Cory. A young college woman with a high school boyfriend found themselves with an unplanned pregnancy. They knew all the options. They had several to choose from. But the one thing they had no choice about was their love for this child that was not yet to be born. This young woman just happened to meet Linda Beale, who worked in an OB/GYN's office. Linda just happened to be Julie's sister. At some point, at one of her office visits, the topic of adoption was discussed. One thing led to another and a private adoption was arranged. On June 30th a little girl was born and her biological mother and father spent hours loving this child that they would soon hand over to a new couple whom they had never met and never would.

I spent 3 days in Bedford, running laps around the hospital, wondering what was happening. We knew that they could change their minds, but their love for this child and what was in her best interest, was stronger than their desire to keep her. How difficult it must have been to place her in another couple's family.

Many couples learn that it takes years and thousands of dollars to find a Caucasian, newborn infant, and this beautiful child is just given to us out of nowhere? It had to be a God thing!

What had I done to deserve this? Why did this blessing happen to me? Life's not fair.

One of the nicest things people have ever said to me by people who don't know Cory's story is, "Cory looks just like you."

When Cory has been asked if she'd ever considered trying to find her biological parents, she says, "I've got wonderful parents. I think it would hurt them if I tried to find my birth parents. There's no need." What did I ever do to deserve that?

I ran 28/30 days in June for 181 miles – starting to get sore – surprise.

July 3:   Ken and Micki Lane (attorney and wife) delivered our new daughter Cory to our family.

July: Ran 28/31 days for 152 miles

August 10:   **Mavis 5 Mile Run** – 31:05

August 13:   Ran 3 miles in the morning – adoption court date Cory is officially ours.

August 18:   **Apple Valley Triathlon** – 2:17

September 15:   Ran a 52 mile week

September 29:   Ran a 54 mile week

October 13:   **Columbus Bank One Marathon**

                     Disappointing – 3:30

Nov. – Dec.:   Minimal running

Evaluation:

Coaching meant that I ran very little in November – March – then a build-up of mileage in August - September for a fall marathon. I was still able to run 1280 miles for the year.

1986

Goals:

No written goals

March: Took three months to get to 100 miles – weight is up to 180 lbs.

April: 75 miles – 175 lbs.

May: 125 miles

June 28:   First 8 mile run – better get going

June: 125 miles

July 13:   First 10 mile run

August: 138 miles

September 6:   ***Fredericktown Tomato Show 5 Mile Run*** – 31:55

September: 142 miles – very few weeks over 449 miles

November 16:   ***Columbus Bank One Marathon***

Went out fast and finished in 3:03 – raced well in 40 degree weather – How can I run that fast on this kind of mileage? Great Job!

Evaluation:

Finished 1986 with 1203 miles – surprising marathon finish on weak build-up. Maybe I can still accomplish something special.

1987

Goals:

1)   Qualify for the Boston Marathon
2)   1400 miles
3)   5 Mile Run in 30 minutes
4)   Be running in December

Jan. – April: 247 miles

May 17:   First 30 mile week – 184 lbs.

June 18:   Vacation to California to visit John and Barb Schafer – ran 7 miles past Dodger Stadium

August 9:   First 40 mile week – pain is developing in my hip

August 15:   ***Mavis 5 Mile Run*** – 32:11 on a sore hip

September: Hip and knee pain

Oct. – Dec.:   Minimal running with pain

Evaluation:

Finished 1987 with 1090 miles and no marathons – disappointing year

1988

Goals:

No written goals

March: Assistant Track Coach at Loudonville High School – ran with the team – 108 total miles for March and 189 total miles – weight is 189 lbs.

May 29: First 30 mile week

July 24: First 8 miles

August 14: ***Mavis 5 Mile Run*** – 33:50

August 22: First 40 mile week – 10 mile long run

September: Two 40+ mile weeks

October 29: 49 mile week – 14 mile long run

November 13: ***Columbus Marathon***

3:14:40 - not too bad
Good enough to want to get better

Evaluation:

Good marathon on minimal training – maybe I can get better. Finished the year with 1334 miles

1989

Goals:

1)   Run the Boston Marathon
2)   Run Columbus Marathon under 3:10
3)   1500 miles
4)   Good health

January: Ran more consistently – 100 mile month

February: 30 miles

March: Two 40+ with long run of 14 miles. This is not enough mileage to run well in Boston – I just want to experience it

April 14:   Arrive in Boston

Some good friends, John and Barb Schafer (formerly from California) lived in Boston while John attended Harvard Business School to get his MBA. I realized that the chance to run the Boston Marathon may never come. It seemed like I was always ten minutes behind the required cutoffs. When I ran a 3:00 marathon, the requirement was 2:50. When the requirement was 3:00, I was running 3:10. So I did what a lot of people did, became a "bandit". A bandit is someone who hasn't qualified for the race but just runs the race from the back of the pack.

I planned to stay with my friends for a few days, find some way to get out to Hopkinton (where the race starts), run the race and just walk off the road right before the finish line. Official entrants have transportation provided to the starting area. Fortunately John found transportation for me on a bus from Harvard, which got me to Hopkinton. My goal had always been to run the Boston Marathon.

April 17: **Boston Marathon**

> GREAT EXPERIENCE! 3:35 – *It was very tough to walk around the starting area with my guilty conscience. But pretty soon the starter's gun was heard, and we were off. The crowds were deafening at times. I could hear the roar way off in the distance. Coming down the road through Wellesley College…. WOW! The hills near the 20 mile mark (Heartbreak Hill) were everything I had imagined. Coming down the final stretch was awesome. I thought about all of the history and tradition. I was running in the footsteps of all the great runners of the past. It was something special.*

May – July: Good consistency in running and lifting, but not many long runs – weight is about 175 pounds

August 20: Ran 10 miles in 1:14 in training

September: Starting to run with Tom Nagy - runs move up to 12 – 13 miles

October 8: Ran 50 mile week with a 14 mile long run
Ran three weeks of 40+ miles but no runs longer than 16 miles

November 12: **Columbus Marathon**

> 3:15 – very disappointing – wanted to actually qualify for Boston so I could "earn" a Boston Marathon medal

Evaluation:

> I finished the year with 1566 miles – not bad
> Will I ever figure out that maybe I should run more long runs?
> I think I'm afraid of the long run.

1990

Goals:
1) 1500 miles
2) Qualify for the Boston Marathon
3) Be running in December

My personal life situation has changed once again. I moved my teaching and coaching back to Mount Vernon High School where I became the JV girls' basketball coach. I now had a lot more time to run (notice the difference in August – October)

January: 110 miles – weight is 180 pounds

February: 93 miles

March: 131 miles

April: 142 miles

May: Ran 30/31 days – 175 mile month – getting into high mileage – running a lot with Tom Nagy – weight 175 pounds

June: 169 miles

July: Vacation in Colorado

July 9:   Ran 6 miles on Great Sand Dunes in Colorado at altitude and I thought my heart was going to come out of my chest. It was like the last 6 miles of the marathon. Received my NYC Marathon Acceptance – better get working with Tom Nagy – weight is 176 pounds.

One needs to understand how the NYC Marathon thing works. It has many more applicants than it can safely manage. Everyone doesn't get in. Eventually it went to a lottery system, but all things weren't equal. There are certain demographics it wants in the race. This lottery system would have a major impact on future NYC Marathons I would enter. That is why I was so excited to have been accepted.

In later years anyone who didn't gain entrance into the NYC Marathon through the lottery could still obtain admissions by becoming a member of one of about 200 charities. If a person joined the charity and raised a required amount of funds for that organization (usually around $2,500), one could obtain entry into the marathon. The Michael J. Fox Foundation for Parkinson's Research was one of those charities that allowed me admission in future years.

August:	191 miles – WOW!
Sept. – Oct.:	47 mile week (long run of 12), 32 mile week (long run of 12), 46 mile week - (2 long runs of 11), 44 mile week (long run of 14), 50 mile week (long run of 12) my weight is down to 170 – I have never worked so hard for this long a time.

November 4: ***New York City Marathon***

Great experience – the crowds were unbelievable –ran an evenly paced race although slow – one can't run in that type of crowd with an expectation of finishing fast – finished in 3:45 - Great Event!

December: Ran a lot more in December than in previous years.

Evaluation:

I finished the year with 1701 miles. Good job – What's next?

1991

Goals:
1)   1700 miles
2)   Qualify for Boston Marathon
3)   Weigh 170 pounds
4)   Be running in December

> *I became the head girls' basketball coach at Mount Vernon High School in the fall of 1991. My weight is about 185 pounds.*

January:	Deep snow – tried running on a small trampoline. Surprising how much of a workout I can get if I put in the time. 135 miles in January
March:	Three runs of 8 – 9 miles
April 10:	Groin is painful – found a lump in my groin
April 19:	Hernia repair surgery – no running for over a month
July:	Incorporated Nautilus Weight Training several days a week
July 21:	Ran 11 miles with Tom Nagy – 39 miles for the week – 164 miles for July
August 10:	**Mavis 5 Mile Run** – 34:00 5 straight 40+ weeks (long run of 11 miles)
September 7:	**Fredericktown Tomato Show 5 Mile Run** – 34:22
September:	Started to use other aerobic machines like elliptical machine instead of running
September 29:	14 miles on the bike path with Tom Nagy
October 3:	While running past the Nazarene University at night, I stepped on a walnut and severely sprained my ankle - discolored – can't sit out too long.

October 25:   48 mile week, with long run of 11 miles

November 3:   15 mile depletion run

November 10:   ***Columbus Marathon***
                   DNF (did not finish) at 14 miles (sick)

Not a good feeling to drop out of a race especially after all the training. Even if it is justified, it makes it easier to do it the next time I am uncomfortable in a marathon. The fact that the course crossed the starting and ending area at 14 miles makes it an easy escape. I think that my mind may have been thinking about the upcoming basketball season instead of this run. I am probably just making an excuse.

Evaluation:

Finished with 1393 miles – not a real good year – weigh 180 lbs.

1992

Goals:
1)   Qualify for the Boston Marathon
2)   Run the NYC Marathon
3)   1800 miles
4)   Weigh 170 pounds
5)   Be running in December

Jan. – March: Using a trampoline to run indoors, nautilus training, elliptical trainer, bike, and treadmill at YMCA

May 6 – 25:   Ran 20 straight days – longest run is 11 miles

June 29 - July 2: Ran at altitude in Albuquerque NM, ran the rim of the Grand Canyon, spent the next week in Mission Viejo, CA. with Schafers, two days of running at Rocky Mountain National Park

July: Discovered another hernia
Ran 119 miles the three weeks between discovering the hernia and surgery

August 7:   Hernia repair surgery
Week 1: 1 mile
Week 2: 20 miles
Week 3: 39 miles
Week 4: 43 miles (long runs of 11 and 12 miles)

September 10:   Shin is painful – very sore – probably returned too fast – YOU THINK?

October 17:   52 mile week with 11 and 12 mile runs

November 1:   ***NYC Marathon***

Upset stomach – two pit stops – got separated from Tom Nagy at 8 mile mark. Finished in 3:49:33 – WOW!

Evaluation:

Ran 1400 miles – I am having more and more setbacks

1993

Goals:
1)   Boston Marathon qualifier – 3:20
2)   Bank One Marathon
3)   Be running in December

Jan. – Feb.:   Slow start because of basketball - 65 miles in two months

March 24:   Sciatic pain
                Alternative workouts cannot replace what you miss

May 1:   First 30 mile week   - try to replace running with other
                forms of exercise (doesn't work) I started to run with
                Don Muncie (also wants to qualify for Boston)

June 1:   40 mile week with long run on bike path of 12 miles with
                Don – integrating hill workouts

June 20:   14 miles with Tom Nagy and Don Muncie – I feel like
                we have a case of "two's company…three's a crowd."

June – July: Running a lot on a treadmill – a more controlled workout

August 5:   Grand Tetons National Park – ran 25 miles at altitude

August 22:   52 mile week – long run of 16 miles with Tom and Don

September 4:   22 mile run with Tom and Don – took 3:05 – longest
                training run – 48 mile week

October 24:   ***Columbus Bank One Marathon***

                2nd time in a row – DNF - retired at mile 13
                No motivation – I knew it would get easier to quit
                It can become a bad habit.

Evaluation:

        Finished the year with 1239 miles - disappointing
        Weight is about 190 pounds

1994

Goals:
1) Complete a marathon again
2) 1200 miles
3) Weigh 180 pounds

It is amazing how much I am lowering my goals. Side note: Things are not going well with Mount Vernon High School girls' basketball team.

Jan. – March: 189 total miles

June 5: Great week of 47 miles – Don Muncie and I are training hard to make each other better and both hope to qualify for the Boston Marathon

July 16: 52 mile week (two 11 mile runs)

July 17: Ran 14 miler – another 52 mile week

August 13: **Precast 5 Mile Run**
Used to be the Mavis 5 Mile Run – finished in 36:10 Gone are the days of trying to run 5 miles in 30 minutes.

August 20: 53 mile week (two 11 mile runs)

August 27: 48 miles (two 11 mile runs and a 9 mile run)

September 3: 53 miles (long run of 13 miles) – hip getting sore – I wonder why?

October 8: 50 mile week (long run of 13 miles)

October 15: 52 mile week (two runs of 11 miles) – hip getting really sore – probably overtraining

October 23: 53 mile week (long runs of 12 and 15 miles

October 30: 56 miles
Great couple of months – two week taper

November 13:   ***Columbus Marathon***

        3:57:20 – good first half, but then???
        All that work!

Evaluation

        What's happening to me?
        I should have run so much faster on this type of mileage
        Good yearly distance of 1818 miles

1995

Goals:

1)   1800 miles
2)   3 marathons including the NYC Marathon
3)   Qualify for Boston (3:20 is needed)
4)   Weigh 175 pounds
5)   Become a better runner

I am no longer coaching basketball – more time

January 21:   20 mile run on the bike path with Don Muncie – the last 8 miles were the "survival shuffle". Good start for the New Year – need more long runs like this 50 mile week in January

February 12:   ***15 mile race in Pickerington***
Zero degrees wind chill (2:01) – crazy race

February 19:   49 mile week (long run of 16 miles)
Really working hard with Don to qualify together for Boston

March 5:   52 mile week with long run of 19 mile

April 2:   ***Athens Marathon in Athens, Ohio***

3:47 what is happening?
Strong first half – very disappointing!

April 23:   53 mile week – long run of 20 miles on bike path with Don - Doing a lot of interval work – 440s @ 7:15 – 7:30 pace

May 14:   ***Cleveland Revco Marathon***

3:28 – good preparation – good nutrition – carbo-loading – I'm back in the game – I just have to shave 8 minutes

July 9:   54 mile week with long run of 15 miles

July 22:   Ran 17 miles on bike path with Don Muncie (2:38)
             52 mile week

July 29:   Ran 19 miles on the bike path (3:09) – really working
             hard with weights, other aerobic machines, treadmills,
             tempo runs (4 miles @ 7:27 pace) – 56 mile week
             211 miles in July - WOW that's working!

August 27:   54 mile week with long runs of 14 and 10 miles

September 3: 19 mile run on bike path with Don (3:00)

September 9: ***Fredericktown Tomato Show 5 Mile Run*** – 35:10

September 24: 54 mile week – long run of 22 miles with Don - hip is
             starting to hurt
             Over training???

September 28: Intervals: 7 x 1 miles @ 7:10 pace (best ever) - hip
             getting sore
             Tried whirlpool and rest and cross training for sore hip

October 7:   12 miles on the bike path – feel crippled
             Several weeks of alternative workouts and chiropractor

November 6: Bone scan shows stress fracture in hip – need to use
             crutches

November 12: ***Columbus Marathon***

             I stand on crutches and cheer Don Muncie as he finishes
             in 3:18 and qualifies for Boston Marathon.

             *I was very happy for Don. He had worked very hard...we had
             worked very hard for this. Maybe I would have qualified with
             Don....who knows?*
             Maybe some things aren't meant to be.

Evaluation:

             Tough year – trained harder – Ran 1729 miles - stress fracture
             No Boston Marathon in 1996

1996

Goals:
1)   Train like an athlete
2)   Run two marathons
3)   1500 miles
4)   Be running healthy in December

January 8:   First jog in three months
                10 minutes on a treadmill – jog ½ mile
                Continued to cross train for several weeks

February 25:   First 5 mile run

March 7:   First 6 mile run
                Butt and hip getting sore again – be careful

April 14:   Weight at 200 pounds – WOW!

May 25:   Ran 10 miles with Don on bike path (9:00 - 9:30/mile)

June 8:   Ran 12 miles on the bike path

June 22:   Ran 14 miles on the bike path – poor run

July 6:   Ran 16 miles on the bike path with Don – increasing
                long runs by 2 miles every other week (38 mile week)

July 20:   Ran 18 miles on the bike path with Don - starting to run
                long but less total miles

August 3:   Ran 20 miles on the bike path with Don

August 10:   ***Precast 5 Mile Run*** - 37:06 – solid run

August 19:   Ran 22 miles with Don - 47 mile week

August 31:   Ran 24 miles on the bike path with Don – Julie biked
                part of it with us – 45 miles on four days

October 5:   Ran 22 miles with Don – last long run – feel strong - 5
                runs of 20 + miles

October 19:   Ran 12 miles on the bike path @ 8:10 pace

November 3:   *NYC Marathon*

                 Ran with Don (4:05) Maybe this is as good as it will get?

Evaluation:

                 Not a bad year overall coming back from a stress fracture.
                 I ran 1349 miles.
                 The window of opportunity to run "well" is getting smaller.

1997

Goals:
1)   Enjoy running
2)   Two Marathons
3)   Qualify for Boston (qualifying time now 3:20)
4)   1500 miles
5)   Stay injury free

January 4:   Start the new year with 14 miles on the bike path – went too fast and body is too fragile – three 40+ mile weeks in January good running

February 22:   Ran 16 miles

March 18:   Ran 18 miles on the bike path by myself

March 20:   Ran 20 miles with Don on the bike path – great run
I can't believe the miles I am doing in March
I want to keep working on some speed work

March 31:   Treadmill workouts – 9 Yazzos - 880s @ 3:25 with a 3:25 rest interval (use 3:25 because I want to run the marathon in 3:25:00)

April 3:   Ran 11 miles on the bike At Marathon Pace (AMP) - 7:30 pace

April 5:   Ran 22 miles with Don on the bike path – solid run in 3:40 – 52 mile week

April 7:   10 Yazzos – tough workout on treadmill

April 12:   Ran 13 miles on bike path AMP

April 29:   Ran 24 miles in 3:55 – last long run

May 4:   ***Cleveland Revco Marathon***

     3:30:25 - I was in the game with 3 miles to go - good run

June-July: Slow buildup with lots of confidence

August 9:   ***Precast 5 Mile Run*** – 36:49 – not much speed

September 13:   Ran 18 miles on the bike path – not increasing too fast

September 27:   Ran 20 miles on the bike path

October 11:   Ran 22 miles on the bike path – SOLO – courage

October 25:   Ran 25 miles on the bike path with Bill Ernst – longest training run ever – 53 mile week

November 9:   ***Columbus Marathon***

3:43 – tried for 3:25 qualifying time

December: Ran a 12 mile run and an 18 mile run – hurt my heel (plantar fasciitis)

Evaluation:

Very frustrated – trained hard all year.
I ran two marathons and 1816 miles.
What more can I do? I don't have any answers.
I just have questions and doubts.

What Has Happened To My Running?

1998

Goals:
1)   Run healthy
2)   1200 miles
3)   Run a marathon under 3:30
4)   Qualify for Boston

January: Heel pain – can't just run through this – try cross training – stationary bike

February 7:   Got orthotic device made (molded to foot for shoe insert) hope that it works

February 28:   10 miles on the bike path – knees getting sore – probably pushing it too much

April: Have run 22 miles so far this year

May 14:   Ran 8 miles on bike path with Don Muncie – wore me out – hip is getting sore

June: A lot of cross training including biking and swimming - not much running

July: Rested for three weeks – some on crutches – no stress facture

Aug. – Dec.:   Battled injuries the rest of the year

Evaluation:

> Wasted year – nothing but fighting injuries
> I ran 551 miles for the year
> Is this all worth it? Why go through all this effort?
> Weight about 195 – 200 pounds

1999

Goals:
1) Keep running pain free
2) Run one marathon
3) Become a master swimmer
4) Weigh 185 pounds

I still want "it" but it seems like I just keep lowering my goals and getting away from what it takes to get it done.

Cory was on the YMCA swim team and at her practices I saw there were some adults going through swim training with the idea of swimming in Master's swim meets. I thought it might be fun. It was fun.

January: I did a lot of swimming at Kenyon (YMCA master's swimming) – ran and walked on the treadmill

February 6: ***Miami University Mardi Gras Master's Swim Meet***
50 Breast: 47.3
100 Breast: 1:27
200 Breast: 2:27
50 Free: 31.5

March: Started to train with heart rate monitor – worked out at certain intensity levels

May: Have only 300 miles for the year

June 5: Ran 12 miles on the bike path – first 30 + mile week

June 25: Ran 14 miles on the bike path with Teri Pokosh – groggy – 38 mile week

July-Aug: Did a lot of treadmill work

August 14: ***Precast 5 Mile*** Race – 40:50
First 40 mile week

August 21: Ran 16 miles on bike path – solo – easy (2:15)

September 18:   Ran 18 miles on bike path – solo – didn't go very well
September 30:   Ran 20 miles on bike path – steady (3:25)

October 31:   Ran 22 miles on bike path – strong (3:42) – 49 mile week
I have gotten some good miles in, now just taper - Three
week taper of 30+ weeks

November 14:   ***Columbus Marathon***

4:57:32 AWFUL!
Got sick at 15 mile mark and had nothing left
Evaluation:

I don't know what is wrong with me. It probably doesn't matter. It just doesn't appear to be worth it. I'm doing everything I can as far as training and I run a marathon in almost 5 hours. This is embarrassing. I'll keep running to maintain health, but **I'll never run a marathon again.** *It's just too much work for that kind of result. I've had my day in the sun when I wasn't too bad a runner, maybe I was pretty good, I don't know. All I know is that I don't want to work that hard for this type of results.*

I did run a total of 1313 miles in 1999.
I'm done with marathons!

2000

Goals:
1)   Be running in December
2)   Run 1200 miles
3)   Have fun

> *I have become the assistant women's basketball coach at Kenyon College. I put a lot of time into helping them be successful. I guess my running life has come to just trying to stay in some type of shape, if I can even maintain that while coaching.*

Jan. – April: Just never got going seriously

May 13:   First 30 mile week

May 22:   First 8 mile run (1:19)

July 7:   First 10 mile run (1:38)

July 21:   First 12 mile run with Teri Pokash

August 3:   Ran 14 mile run with Teri Pokash

August 12:   ***Precast 5 Mile Run*** – 44 minutes

August 17:   Ran 16 miles – solo (2:45)

Evaluation:

No marathons – 983 miles for the year

2001

Goals:

No written goals

Jan. – Dec.:   Didn't get much done to stay in any kind of shape – 715
miles

*This was the last runner's log that I officially kept. The total miles
for all years were 32,473 miles. There were many more miles run
after 2001, but somehow they didn't seem worth writing down.
Who knows what the future has in store. It has been an interesting
journey…some good…some bad. It's made me a better person. It
changed my life.*

Are You Sure That You Want to Know?

Sometimes a person has a question, but one has to be careful about whether he/she really wants to know the answer. That's how I felt in the early 2000s. I knew that I wasn't running as well as in the past, but didn't know if I needed to change something in my training or if there was some other reason. My wife thought I was just getting old. It couldn't be that. Being 50 years old might make a difference, but I felt that it was something else.

I remember running with Tom Nagy out by the high school. I was telling him that I felt that something was wrong with me, that my legs just didn't feel like they had in the past.

"Maybe you're just getting older," was his first his response.

I asked him if he had been talking to my wife. "It's more than that. When we get done with this run and I take a shower, my left hand won't function the way it should. And I find myself leaning against the shower wall to maintain my balance."

He stated, "Maybe you should go see a doctor."

But a guy like me doesn't go see a doctor for something like that…at least not right away. As I continued to analyze my running and overall condition, I decided to seek some medical advice. I first went to my general practitioner, Dr. Larry Reed in Mount Vernon. After his evaluation of my situation, he said that I should see a specialist in Columbus, at the Madden Center for Movement Disorders, which is part of The Ohio State Medical Center.

I met a woman who would have a major impact on my life for the next decade. Dr. Sandra Kostyk was a neurologist and a specialist in Parkinson's disease and Huntington's disease.

I liked her from day one. She was about my age and was, in my opinion, a genius. She was sort of quirky, but I had the utmost respect for her. Over the years, we spent a lot of time discussing parenting. She often asked me for advice for her teenage sons.

After a series of neurological tests, many of which seemed like what police do when they test for a DUI, she offered her diagnosis. She said, "Matt, you have Parkinson's Disease…the disease that afflicts Michael J. Fox and Mohamed Ali."

Her words weren't completely surprising to hear. As I sat in the room waiting for her to arrive (I would later learn that waiting for her was normal), I read the posters with Parkinson's symptoms and I just kept saying, "Yep, I've got that one, and that one and that one." My first question was, "Well, what do we do to fix this?"

Her response was not entirely what I wanted to hear. "There is no cure. You don't show serious symptoms right now. With proper medication, we may be able to delay the progression of the disease. But you need to know that Parkinson's is a progressive degenerative disease which as of today has no cure."

Progressive and degenerative…to me that meant I was never going to get any better than I was at that moment. This is as good as it gets. I decided right then that this thing was just an inconvenience and I wasn't going to let this thing consume me. Maybe I was in denial. She tried to assure me that medications were continually improving and they were able to delay the progression of the disease. But she said that the best things were having a good attitude, staying active and exercising. I could do that. I was a runner.

Dr. Kostyk told me that some of her patients were able to live a relatively normal lifestyle, but that I might want to see what kind of disability insurance plan I had. My symptoms were minimal. I did not have the tremors in the hands or fingers. I did have some rigidity and lack of flexibility. There was awkwardness to my walking gait. I felt like when I walked, especially when in a crowded space like a hallway, that it was like I was walking on a moving bus. I just didn't feel balanced. My left arm didn't swing when I walked. I had heard some students whisper that I looked like Frankenstein. It is a symptom called "masking". It's when the muscles in your face are relaxed and drawn. My voice was soft and my handwriting almost impossible to read. Writing in a checkbook, recording grades in a grade book, or writing on the blackboard was very difficult. Balance was a problem, especially getting up out of a chair or off the floor. Turning around and changing directions were minor problems. There was a period of time when I would find myself walking faster and faster, like I was walking downhill. I also lost my sense of smell. I just considered all of these to be an inconvenience.

At the end of the first session, Dr. Kostyk told me to go home and think about how I was going to approach the future. We would discuss a plan of action from a medication standpoint as well as from a psychological perspective at our second meeting in a month. She wanted to look into an ongoing double blind research study that might meet my needs and allow me to help in Parkinson's research.

The first thing I did that day after leaving her office was to go to a bookstore and purchase Michael J. Fox's book *Lucky Man*. Michael is eight years younger than me and had publically come forward with his diagnosis of Parkinson's disease. In his book he talked about his journey and how he handled his situation. I recognized a lot of my feelings expressed in that book.

One of the first decisions I had to make after being diagnosed was to decide how and when and to whom I was going to tell of my misfortune. I selfishly wanted to hold onto the information for a while. I guess I felt that I had no control of the fact that I had this disease; I ought to have some control about the way it was going to be told to the public. But what good does it do to keep this thing between my wife and me? I realized that there was nothing to be gained by keeping it secret. This was who I was now. But once it's out there, there's no getting it back. I started with my family and then my immediate group of friends. I wanted as many as possible to hear it from me instead of from someone else. Most were concerned because they only knew the common view of Parkinson's as some person, probably in a wheel chair, who is shaking a lot and can't control his motions. I know that was the view I had. Many assumed I was in a certain amount of pain or that I had been given a death sentence. I felt that the more I remained calm and didn't overreact to this news, the more comfortable others soon became.

When I returned to Dr. Kostyk's office the next month, I told her that right now this was just an inconvenience. I had to deal with it and I wasn't going to be consumed by this thing. I would face the challenges before me as they came...not before. She entered me in a double blind study on a dopamine agonist that was administered from a transdermal patch, placed on the skin, instead of taking the drug orally. There was a certain titration period where I came to her office each week and received new patches at a higher dose. I also received EKGs and blood testings free of charge, as well as observations by the doctors and staff. Neither the doctor nor I was supposed to know if I was receiving a placebo or the real drug. It didn't take me long to realize that I had the drug because my body reacted by becoming nauseous almost immediately upon moving to a new dose. Some weeks I couldn't get home from Columbus without pulling the car over and vomiting. Fortunately it only lasted a day or two. I was part of a two year study and then at the end of two years, I was allowed to continue taking it for free until the FDA made a decision and the study was complete. When the FDA finally approved the drug, something went wrong with how it was originally produced and I could no longer take the drug. I thought the general idea of a one-a-day patch was very efficient for me. I didn't have to remember all the times that I had to take medications.

After the study, I was basically put on drugs taken orally, some of which I took previously in addition to the patches. Stalevo, Azilect, Requip XL, and Amantadene became a daily routine for me. This combination seemed to work well for me. Most doctors will tell you that they are just making educated guesses. It is basically a crap shoot with continual tweaking until they find what works best for each patient. I can't emphasize enough the benefit my running has had as an important part of my plan. It may be the most important part of my trying to control the degenerative process.

What did I do when I taught school? I tried to pretend it didn't change my ability to teach and just acted like it didn't make a difference. But eventually I took advantage of available technologies. I started to use power point presentations to avoid having to write on the board. The school also provided audiology equipment in my room, which created a kind of surround sound effect. It helped amplify my soft voice.

After a year or two, I decided that I would begin the year by telling my students right away. On the first day of class, I produced a power point presentation, stating the standards for the class, the way the class would be run and so forth. I gave them some personal information about myself, my family, and my interests. It was an exciting first day power point, including music to go along with the slides. There was a slide with a picture of Michael J. Fox and Mohamed Ali and the question, "How many of you know these two men?" This was followed by first day giggles in response to the question. Someone would always say "I know them." On the next slide I asked the question, "What does Mr. Wilbur have in common with these two men?" Now the giggling had started to quiet down because they weren't quite sure where this was going. The next slide said, "We all have Parkinson's disease." Now the whole class was silent, respectful and attentive as the following slides basically talked about the disease, how it affected me, what my symptoms were, what they could expect from me, and what I expected from them. I think my openness to discuss my situation made them a lot more sensitive. I heard very few jokes that high school kids have a tendency to make when they make uneducated judgments about people who are a little bit different.

I spent several years worrying about how my future might look. As I approached the end of my career, I made a change in direction with which I was going to live with Parkinson's. I was 56 years old and I decided that wherever Parkinson's was going to lead me in the future, my life had already been blessed beyond measure. I had received things that I never earned or deserved. People had done things for me that I never could pay back. Maybe it was time for me to pay it forward. But how?

Journey to the Finish Line

In the spring of 2009, I had been running fairly consistently when my daughter Kristen Martin called me and said, "Dad, there is an event going on here in Cincinnati this weekend called the Flying Pig. It has races of all distances: the 5K, 10K, half marathon and the marathon. Why don't you come down and run a 5K? I know you've been running some. You used to say that anyone could run a 5K. It's only 3.1 miles."

I replied that I hadn't run a race of any distance in over ten years, but that I would think about it. The more I thought about it, the more I realized that we were going to go down from Mount Vernon to watch her run anyway, so I thought, "Maybe I'll do this."

So as we drove to Cincinnati on Friday, I called her and said, "If you can get me registered by tomorrow, I'll run. But I don't want to run the 5K; I want to run the 10K." I figured it would be easier to run 6.2 miles with a thousand other people than by myself. I was going to just treat it like a training run. I didn't think much about it until I stepped off the sidewalk and into the street. Then it all came rushing back to me: the feeling of being in the arena with other athletes, the feeling of getting energy from the person next to you, and you're giving energy to them, the feeling of sweat and exertion, the feeling of setting goals and going after them, the feeling of having doubts and overcoming them, and the feeling of taking on something that is difficult and achieving it.

When I finished that race, my legs were moving really slowly, but my mind was in a full sprint. It was talking to me like a crazy man. Saying things like, "Wow, I can't believe how great that feels. Could I do that again real soon? Do you think I could run a marathon again? Would I even want to run a marathon, knowing I couldn't run it in 5, 6 or maybe 7 hours? Maybe I couldn't run it at all. Maybe I could run for a cause. Maybe I could take these bad cards I'd been dealt and do something good. Maybe I could pay it forward."

I went to the Michael J. Fox website and saw that there was a group of people called Team Fox. Team Fox (which began in 2006) was a group of about 1500 active men and women who were committed to raising funds and awareness for Parkinson's research through the Michael J. Fox Foundation for Parkinson's Research. Team Fox has raised approximately $5 million for the Fox Foundation. They raised money in a variety of ways: golf outings, gala events, garage sales, climbing mountains and participating in athletic events. They took whatever they had a passion for and tried to turn it into a fundraising event. I decided to raise money by asking friends and family to sponsor me, and I would run the 2009 New York City Marathon on November 7, 2009.

The marathon was very special for several reasons. My older daughter, Kristen Martin, who had become a good marathon runner after marriage (sub 4:00 marathon), said she'd run the whole marathon with me. My whole family got to go to New York City that weekend. My wife Julie, my other daughter Cory Wilbur, my son-in-law Jeff Martin and my two granddaughters, Ava (age 3) and Grace (age 1) were all there to support Kristen and me. The weekend was somewhat bitter sweet, because my mom passed away a month before the marathon. Her journey on this earth was now complete.

The Team Fox marathon team had an opportunity to meet one another on Saturday night at a pre-race dinner put on by Team Fox. All of those in the room had some type of an association with someone who had Parkinson's. Maybe it was a parent, grandparent, friend or co-worker that had the disease and they all wanted to help find a cure. Out of the two hundred Team Fox runners, there were three or four of us who actually were running with Parkinson's disease. The highlight of the evening was having Michael J. Fox speak to us and if you were lucky, you might have had a chance to speak to him on a personal level. I was one of the lucky ones.

The first Sunday in November is something special in New York City. Kristen and I woke up at 4:00 am and got our things together that we would need for the day ahead. Because of security concerns, everything we took had to be put in a clear tote bag they provided for us. We were excited but tried to conserve energy, as we took a cab from our hotel to where we would pick up our Team Fox busses which would take us to Staten Island. We boarded the busses at 5:00 am, departed at 5:30 am and arrived at the starting area around 6:00 am. There was a certain degree of team camaraderie, despite the fact that we were basically strangers.

When we arrived at the starting area, we entered a wave of people all getting off hundreds of busses. Everyone who is entered in the race is given a prearranged method by which they get to Staten Island. Most come by bus, but some come on the Staten Island Ferry.

The best description of the starting area is it was like a refugee camp. Forty-five thousand runners are waiting for a race to start. There are three areas that runners are assigned to: orange group, blue group and a green group. Everybody is divided based on one's projected finish time. We find a piece of real estate and lie down and rest for the next few hours. There are bagels, energy bars, water and energy drinks available to top off our glycogen levels and be fully hydrated before we leave. We also try to coordinate going to one of the hundreds of Porta-potties. We would like to go right before we leave, but everybody else has the same idea, so we have to wait in a line of maybe ten to fifteen people.

The race starts in three waves: one leaving at 11:00 am, the second wave leaves at 11:20 am and the third wave departs at 11:40 am. Each wave has about thirty corrals in which we report before our wave is taken onto the Verrazano Bridge. There are also three starting areas on the bridge: the top right side, the top left side and the lower level of the bridge. Because of the staggered starts, a computer chip is placed on our shoe laces (now on our number bib) so they can scan us as we go by certain check points and can give us our exact finish time.

The beginning of the race is very crowded but it starts to thin out by the end of the bridge, which is about at the 2 mile mark. We are then on our journey that will take several hours, taking us into Brooklyn, Queens, into Manhattan on 1st Avenue, where the crowds are unbelievable, into the Bronx and finally back to Manhattan coming down 5th Avenue. Michael J. Fox lives on Fifth Avenue at about mile 23. He spent much of the day greeting Team Fox runners as they went by. We turn into Central Park, thinking we're almost done, but we still have a few miles to go before the finish line and we receive our medals. One of the most difficult things to do is to find our way out of the park and to locate our family.

Kristen brought a camera to document the events of the weekend including the race. I think she was hoping to get a picture of Michael J. Fox. Which she did! Upon completing the marathon in a time of just over 7 hours, we went to a post-race Team Fox gathering and couldn't believe how many people told us how we were such an inspiration for having finished the race. It was almost embarrassing. One young man came up to me and said, "Matt, I ate the pre-race dinner with you last night and I didn't know you had Parkinson's. I can't tell you how inspiring it is that you and your daughter finished the race."

I replied, "I appreciate what you are saying, but I've run twenty-five marathons and I know that a 7 hour marathon shouldn't inspire anyone."

"I don't think you understand," he replied. "My father has Parkinson's and for him and others like him, just getting through the day is like running a marathon."

When we returned to Ohio, I asked Kristen if she would put her images on the computer. I wanted to make a short music video or slide show for her to thank her for running with me. I didn't realize that she was doing the same thing for me. It took me fifteen hours to make ten minutes of video. Kristen on the other hand is a professional wedding videographer and was able to produce about twenty minutes of video. So within a month, I had two videos, both taken from the same material, but from two different perspectives. I asked myself, "What if I put these two videos back to back on one dvd? I wonder how it would turn out." I believe that somehow God took my story about how I got involved with Team Fox, the pictures, images, video and music and put it all together in such a way as to have an impact on thousands of lives. We made approximately eight hundred copies of our dvd, which we titled, "Journey to the Finish Line" and gave it to whomever we thought would enjoy watching it at home with family and friends.

I told people that there were three things I wanted viewers to get from watching this video: 1) to understand my story and why and how I got involved with Team Fox, 2) to see what it was like to be involved with an event the size and magnitude of the New York City Marathon, and 3) to understand the value of family. To have Kristen run the whole NYC Marathon with me and get me to the finish line is something I will cherish the rest of my life. I also realize that Ava and Grace were only 3 and 1 at the time, but in a few years they may look at the video and understand why their mom and grandpa ran through the streets of New York that weekend.

When I first decided to run the 2009 NYC Marathon for Team Fox, I had only two goals that I wanted to accomplish: 1) to see if I could run a marathon again at the age of 56, after a ten year absence from the event and having been diagnosed with Parkinson's disease and 2) to see if I could raise the required $2500 necessary to run with the Team Fox NYC Marathon Team. But I soon realized that much more was in store for me than that. That first year with Team Fox, because of the generosity of family and friends, we were able to contribute almost $8000 to the Fox Foundation. But more importantly than that was that I realized that running the NYC Marathon for Team Fox had given me a platform to speak to people of all ages and walks of life, in many different venues, not only how to live with Parkinson's disease, but how one can choose to live with all the "bad" things that come into all of our lives. Because "bad" things happen to everyone...no one is exempt. Maybe "bad" is not the proper word, but there are things that come into our lives that rob us of part of who we are. Maybe it takes some of our health. Maybe it takes some of our relationships or maybe it steals some of our finances. But the one thing it can't take from us is our "attitude". That's ours to keep. And the nice part about it is that we can make it whatever we want it to be.

It wasn't long after speaking to these groups that people started to use the word "inspiration" and directing it my way. They said that I was an inspiration. I was never comfortable with the word. How could someone who ran a 7 hour marathon be an inspiration to anyone? I wasn't an inspiration!

Shortly after making the dvd, I gave my students the kind of day every student wants to have. We didn't do any math and just watched the video and talked about what they thought of it and what it had meant to me to be involved with Team Fox. I went home and told Julie that this is probably why the public schools get such a bad reputation. All we do is watch videos that have no value and don't have anything to do with mathematics. I had wasted the tax payer's money. I told her I hoped to make it up in the near future.

Sure enough, the next day there was an envelope on my desk with my name on it. Teachers don't like to see things like that on our desks because it is either from an angry parent or an administrator who doesn't like something we've done. I opened the envelope and it was from one of my students, a senior in one of my pre-calculus classes. I'll call her Brittanie, because her name was Brittanie. This is what it said:

Mr. Wilbur:

Congratulations of a great run and raising an amazing amount of money for Team Fox. I wanted to stress how much your story meant to me yesterday. You're incredibly humble for thinking you are not an inspiration, because just a small story completely changed my life yesterday. It is amazing how you view life. Someone who has had so many trials, having so much faith is astounding. My father was a strong Christian and passed away when I was 11. I pulled away from the church, but came back in the 9th grade, and have been going strongly for almost three years, but lately with the stress of school and life, my faith has been a little rocky. A sentence you said yesterday really struck me. You said, "If you're not living for something, you're probably dying." I spent the rest of the day finding different ways to live my life, different things to live for. From just one sentence, I made a complete 180. I decided I need to strengthen many relationships in my life. I need to be a better daughter, a better sister, a better student, and a better friend. I need to strengthen my relationship with God and to be the person my dad would be proud of. I want to thank you for touching my heart and rekindling my spirit. Thank you for helping me remember to live for something instead of slowly dying. I'm incredibly appreciative for who you are and for everything you're doing.

God Bless,
Brittanie

After reading that letter, I said to myself, "If that is what an inspiration looks like, if that's what it means, then I'm willing to be one. If my running the NYC Marathon for Team Fox can somehow touch the heart and spirit of another human being, the species that I happen to belong to, then I ought to continue to run."

So I decided to run the 2010 NYC Marathon. This time Kristen was going to run with me as a member of Team Fox. I knew that whatever shape I was in, Kristen could get me to the finish line. But about four weeks before the marathon, she told me that she couldn't go to NYC with me. She and the rest of my family were going to Colombia, South America for about a month, to meet and adopt two young boys, Victor (age 14) and Jesus (age 9), who would soon be my grandsons. Although that was a neat thing, it meant that I was now going to have to run the marathon by myself. I hadn't trained for that. I knew from past marathons what it took to run by myself and I hadn't come close. I knew that I couldn't cheat the marathon. If I don't put in the miles, it will eat me up and make a coward out of anyone. I didn't think I could run the race by myself.

So the Saturday night before the race, I had a little talk with God and said, "I know that you have been involved in this journey from the beginning and that you wanted me to use this as a platform to speak to people about keeping a positive attitude when "bad" things happen. But you also know that I haven't trained properly for this marathon and I am not sure if I can run this by myself. If you want me to continue on this journey I've been on, you're going to have to give me some help."

The next morning I reported to the Team Fox busses at 5:00 am for a 5:30 am departure to the starting line. I sat on my seat wondering how I was going to be able to run alone…as if running with 45,000 other runners could be considered running by myself. About five minutes before we were to leave, a Team Fox leader came onto our bus and asked, "Is Matt Wilbur on this bus?" That startled me a bit since it was 5:30 am on a Sunday in downtown Manhattan.

"That would be me," I said.

"There is someone on the sidewalk that would like to speak to you."

A young man stepped up on the bus, walked back to my seat, shook my hand and said, "I'm Mike Dubin from Ann Arbor, Michigan. You probably don't remember me, but I met you last year after you and your daughter finished the marathon. I told you that I was so inspired that you had finished the race because my father had Parkinson's. This is probably a coincidence, but I was assigned by Team Fox to be your daughter's mentor in preparation for this race. We emailed quite a bit over the summer and I realize that she's in South America doing a great thing. I just wanted you to know that and to ask you if you needed someone to run with today."

I couldn't believe it. God had answered my prayer and sent someone that I didn't even know to support me and to see that I got to the finish line, an angel, so to speak. And Mike Dubin started with me in the very back of the third wave of runners, spent 7 ½ hours of his Sunday supporting me, running with me through the streets of New York City and getting me to the finish line.

When I finished the 2010 NYC Marathon, 45,000 runners started the race. About 44,800 runners finished in front of me. I finished in the bottom .4% of all runners. Many have asked why I ran when I was so far from even being considered average. It was a good question. Then I realized that only 2% of all Americans ever run a marathon and only a handful run the NYC Marathon with Parkinson's. I felt that I could be proud of that.

The summer of 2011, I got the chance to go up to Ann Arbor with Julie to have a cookout with Mike and Darla Dubin and Mike's mom and dad, Patti and Howard Dubin. Mike's dad did have Parkinson's pretty badly. Before I left he turned to me with a special smile (as if he knew something I would learn in the future) and said, "Keep fighting." I assured him that I would.

These experiences more than affirmed to me that I was to continue running the NYC Marathon at least for 2011. This was to be my victory lap. I was going to run this with Kristen and Mike, the two people I had run with in 2009 and 2010. Four weeks before the marathon, Mike's dad passed away due to complications from Parkinson's disease. Mike pulled some strings and we were able to start at the back of the first wave of runners, but we still finished in 7:30. It was a joyous day. Howard Dubin was smiling down on us.

In three years I have received over $21,000 in contributions for the Michael J. Fox Foundation. I have been able to speak to many groups of people and talk about keeping a positive attitude when faced with bad circumstances. I was 58 years old. What's next?

I Think I Have a Story to Tell

(MATT'S ATTEMPT AT PUBLIC SPEAKING)

According to *The Book of Lists*, public speaking is the number one fear of people, above even death. I don't know why I thought I had a story worth telling and would be willing to stand in front of hundreds of people…. stand there, by myself, with the chance of embarrassing myself, and take the risk. I think it's a lot like my running….everybody could probably do it, it's simple. There's really no talent involved. The hard part is taking that first step and facing up to my fears of failure. If I have had any success with presentations I've made over the years, I think it's that I portray myself as just an average guy like those who are listening. That's not a hard thing to portray because most of the folks probably know who I am and can attest to that fact. I've never claimed to be something I'm not. The idea that this normal, average, guy, like anyone else, standing up there telling a story, strikes something inside most folks that says "I have to give that guy some credit. He is just like me, but I wouldn't want to be up there. If a guy like that can do something like he's doing, maybe I can do more with my life."

I believe that we all have a story to tell and that people really do like to hear someone honestly talk about one's story. Maybe we find out that everybody has some type of problem and we've been thinking we were the only one. There is a sense of being connected with others. To hear someone reply, "I have a similar situation," immediately gives me a chance to touch the heart and spirit of another human being.

Mayor's Prayer Breakfast

My first serious public speaking opportunity happened in 2002. I had been the "huddle coach" for Mount Vernon High School's Fellowship of Christian Athletes for several years and was asked to be a speaker at Mount Vernon's Mayor's Prayer Breakfast. The breakfast is an annual event where people buy tickets to a breakfast and pray for the governmental officials (only in small town America). They also get to listen to a "big time", well-known figure (possibly a sports figure or politician) and to hear from a local "not so famous or well known, community figure". You can guess which one I was.

I was the lead-in act for Kenneth Blackwell. He was a well-known state politician who had hopes of being governor someday, or maybe even a higher position. I really didn't know what they wanted me to talk about, so I just told the honest story of how FCA began at Mount

Vernon High School - how a handful of students wanted a vehicle in which to share their faith. They needed an adult sponsor (huddle coach) and since I had some previous experience with FCA, we started meeting on Friday mornings at 6:45 am before school.

Any time one has a religious group involved with public schools, there is the issue of separation of church and state. Mount Vernon's FCA was no different. It became a political and legal issue. But calmer heads prevailed and I think we knew where to find a comfortable way for both sides to coexist. The fact that Mount Vernon High School's FCA had grown to one of the largest FCA huddles in the state and even within the entire country, elevated the importance of finding a solution that everyone could accept.

After the ten minutes of delivering a speech that I had prepared for weeks, I (or FCA which I represented) received a standing ovation. I thought, "How did that happen? I am not good enough to deserve that much praise." Maybe God could use an average guy like me to touch people's heart. Maybe if I have an honest story to tell, maintain an honest, humble approach, and have time to prepare…maybe I could do this public speaking gig in the future. As a teacher, I had to stand in front of a class every day. That gives me time to practice. But this kind of speaking is much more intense.

FCA Sports Legends Awards Banquet

My second major speaking engagement involved the 2006 "FCA Sports Legends Awards Banquet". This is a major fundraising event held in a huge restaurant each year in Columbus, to promote and fund FCA within the state of Ohio. Each year they select a "Sports Legend of the Year". This is usually a nationally known sports figure who has been involved with FCA's mission. They then select and recognize a "FCA Huddle Coach of the Year" as well as recognizing Christian student athletes from different schools. I was to receive the "Huddle Coach of the Year Award". Although very honored with the recognition, I was told I was expected to speak for about five minutes.

This was major intensity. No pressure. Just about 500 well-to-do folks deeply involved with FCA, who wanted it to have an impact on the youth of today's schools. This is one of the first times that I realized how pressure could affect my Parkinson's symptoms. My arms were starting to show signs of tremor and my walking was off balance.

The dinner involved going through a buffet line within a huge ballroom and taking it to an assigned seat. I was so worried about the event that I had Julie carry the plate for me. When I sat down, the first thing I did was mentally navigate how I would get through the tables, climb some steps onto a stage, walk across it to a podium, receive an award, speak for five minutes, and then get back to my seat while shaking from Parkinson's.

I remember thinking that not only would I be in front of all these important people, but that my presentation would be displayed on two huge screens, so those in the back could see. When I finally got introduced, I remember having a sense of calm come over me that could only be from God. The shaking went away as I ascended the steps. As I took my first few breaths before beginning my talk, I almost started to laugh. Here I was ten feet above tables that included Heisman Trophy Winner Archie Griffin, Ohio State University Head Football coach Jim Tressell, CBS broadcaster Clark Kellogg, who had just returned from "March Madness", as well as other past and present OSU athletes. I was going to be speaking to them. Wow!

I spoke again of the story of Mount Vernon's FCA and how God had chosen to use a small rural community like Mount Vernon to show what He is still capable of doing and that no one had sent Him a memo about not being allowed in the public schools. Once again my speech was well received.

But even after a great experience like that, God brought me back to reality quickly. I have a friend from Mount Vernon, Bryan Hawkins, who had become involved with the Campus Crusade for Christ (Athletes in Action) at The Ohio State University. He was actively involved with bible studies with members of the coaching staff at OSU.

Bryan Hawkins is also part of my son-in-law, Jeff Martin's (Kristen's husband) extended family. There was a family gathering the week after I spoke. Bryan came up to Kristen and said he had something cool to tell her. He said that the day after I spoke, he was at a bible study with Jim Tressell. Coach Tressell came right up to Bryan and said, "Aren't you from Mount Vernon? I heard this man from Mount Vernon High School's FCA speak last night and he did a fantastic job. We need more men like that."

Kristen's response to Bryan was, "Who is Jim Tressell?"

Knox County GED Graduation

My wife Julie worked for the Knox County Department of Jobs and Family Services and was very involved with helping people of all ages to train for and to receive their GEDs. She had helped hundreds feel the pride of that accomplishment. Well, in the spring of 2009, shortly after deciding to get involved with Team Fox, the head of the county ABLE program was talking to Julie about finding a graduation speaker. Julie asked me whether I'd feel comfortable speaking, and I said absolutely not.

But after some prodding and telling me how well I was getting at public speaking, I consented. Fortunately the graduation director said she had found someone else. I was not upset. Then some days later, she called Julie and said her speaker was not going to work out and would I still be willing to speak. I accepted.

All I could remember from every graduation I'd ever attended was that nobody wanted to hear the graduation speaker. They just wanted to see their loved one walk across the stage, receive the diploma, go to a reception, have some cake and move on. I was going to be that graduation speaker no one wanted to hear. On top of that, the fact that they were in a GED program meant that they had not had a good experience in the public schools. For some reason they had quit or been removed from the system that I was going to represent. Some of these recipients may have been my former students. Maybe some had flunked my class. Maybe I was part of the reason they were in this situation.

The theme for graduation was "A Journey of a Thousand Miles Begins with a Single Step. Go the Distance", which at least meant that I had some connection with the graduation theme. I decided to tell them about my running past and then about my present situation with Parkinson's. I hoped I might get some sympathy, which would ease their hatred for graduation speakers and public school teachers.

As I started to speak, I thought to myself, "These people are actually listening to me." I tried to parallel my running a marathon with going through the educational process. I told them that my worst running experience had been when I looked at the race results, not seeing a slow time, but seeing the letters "DNF"....Did Not Finish, next to my name. For some reason I had dropped out of the race. I could probably justify it. Maybe I felt sick or maybe I was afraid of being injured, but in my heart, I knew quitting had been my decision, and I felt quitting in the future had forever become an easier thing to do. I told them that maybe they could relate. I said my only recourse was to either quit running or find a different course with the same requirement of running 26.2 miles and receive the same praise and honor any other person that completes the course received. We all get the same medal.

It was about at this moment that the crowd all started to applaud. Students and parents were all looking right at me and applauding. My first thought was that they were telling me, "Thank you very much, but we feel you're done now". But that wasn't the case. I finished my talk, was warmly received and it was over…at least for the moment.

After they had their ceremony and transitioned to a reception, many people from varying backgrounds came up and not only thanked me, but told me of people they knew in their lives who were struggling with Parkinson's or some other hardship. I had connected with people I didn't even know. I had touched their hearts and spirits.

For weeks, the graduation director wouldn't stop telling Julie and me how I was the best graduation speaker they had ever had. It was embarrassing. But in my mind, it gave me a certain confidence in knowing that if I was honest with my story and allowed myself to be vulnerable, maybe I could touch someone's life. This had been my first of many testimonies I was to give regarding my Parkinson's experience.

Mount Vernon First Presbyterian Church

Within a month of that graduation, I made a decision that maybe my Parkinson's story was worth sharing with others. It wasn't a sense of conceit, but a sense that someone's life might be touched by my journey. One Sunday morning before church, I told our pastor Jonathon Fettig, of Mount Vernon First Presbyterian Church, that I thought I had something I wanted to share with the congregation. We had a precedent for such a thing within our service called "Minute for Mission" where someone shares a project he/she is involved with and maybe asks for financial support.

Pastor Fettig asked if I had a date in mind. I said October 8th. That was over five months away and four weeks before the NYC Marathon. He said that it would be a Communion Sunday.

I said, "I realize that and what I have to share will relate."

He asked, "How much time do you need?"

"All of it," I replied. "I'll give you a day off and I'll take care of the sermon."

He agreed.

What had I done? We had two services, an early "contemporary" service, and a more "traditional" second service. I wasn't too nervous about speaking at the first service. They were open to new things happening on any particular Sunday. They met in Fellowship Hall and tried to create a more relaxed atmosphere. The second service was made up of some of the pillars of the church. Some wonderful people go to that service. We raised our families together. I went to that service many times. I always sat in the same pew. But the second service is called "traditional" for a reason. Things have been done in a particular, orderly fashion for years. It's worked in the past, let's not change it. There is a certain comfort in knowing what to expect on a Sunday morning. I had been a member of that church for over thirty years and couldn't remember too many times when someone gave the type of testimony I planned to give.

I used all of the five months to prepare for what I wanted to say. I would find myself saying parts of my speech while driving a car. In August I went on a road trip with a friend of mine to The Grand Tetons. For two nights in a row, I could not get the thoughts of my speech out of my head while attempting to sleep. Finally on the third night, when the ideas flooded my mind, I pulled my laptop under my sleeping bag and started to type. I didn't have any trouble sleeping the rest of the trip.

When October rolled around, I knew that what I had prepared was what I really wanted to say. But would I be able to pull it off? Facing people with whom I had shared so much of my life and sharing my story… How would they react?

When I give a talk, I type up what I want to say, but try to know it well enough that I don't need to rely on my notes. I just hold them as a crutch. After being introduced by the pastor, I walked out from behind the pulpit and started telling my story.

I reviewed the chronology of my running history, the highs and the lows. I told them about receiving my diagnosis and deciding that I was not going to let this thing consume me. I mentioned that bad things happen to everyone. I discussed the idea that when some folks look at the "cup" of their life, they see it as half empty and not capable of accomplishing much with their life. Some see the "cup" as half full and there is still plenty left to accomplish and contribute.

One of the concepts I introduced was that when "bad" things come into my life, I look at my "cup" and say, "How can I complain? The cup doesn't belong to me. It's been lent to me for 60, 70 or maybe 80 years. I realized that something had been taken from my cup, that there was some bad stuff in my cup, but there was some good stuff in there also. It was my job to accomplish as much and contribute as much as I could with whatever was in my cup and give glory to God who lent me the cup in the first place."

I then talked about how my daughter, Kristen, who was sitting down front, had asked me to run in Cincinnati during the Flying Pig weekend. I mentioned my reaction to running in an event again, after ten years, and maybe using my running to pay it forward for the blessings I'd received since having been diagnosed with Parkinson's. I talked about my involvement with Team Fox and my plans to run the NYC Marathon in four weeks. I concluded with what I had learned on this journey. I stated that when I look at my cup now, I don't see it as half empty or half full. My life has been blessed beyond measure. I had received so many things that I didn't earn or deserve. People had done so much for me that I couldn't pay back, but maybe I could pay forward. My cup is so full of blessings that it's overflowing and I have to sip them out of the saucer.

I finished and sat down, not wanting to look around. I had looked around during the talk to try to see how they were reacting. I really couldn't tell. They seemed to be paying attention, but maybe they were just putting on their nice faces. Julie asked me later, "Didn't you see and hear all those people crying during your talk?" I had seen my dad in the back, sitting in his wheelchair, crying through the whole talk, but that's just my dad.

While standing at the door as people started to leave the sanctuary, I thought to myself, "Well, they will shake my hand, say I did a nice job, and go to lunch". But one after another, they came up to me visibly shaken. Some hugged me and cried words that were hard to hear. Most were in a state of, "I don't believe what I just heard come from this man we've all known for so long."

I was emotionally fatigued. I had so much to think about. I guess I better finish the race now or this will all be sort of meaningless. Somehow, I had an impact on a lot of people and had touched their hearts, and I hadn't even run the race yet. God was definitely on this journey with me.

Knox County Parkinson's Support Group

In the last week of October, the last week before the marathon, I had an opportunity to speak to a Parkinson's support group that meets each month at Knox Community Hospital. I had gone to a few meetings, and to be honest, didn't feel comfortable. Most of the folks were in their 70s or 80s and had Parkinson symptoms that were quite evident. Most were brought to the meeting by a spouse or caregiver. A good portion of the time was spent talking about symptoms and medications they were taking and when their next doctor's appointment was. God love them, but that environment does nothing but bring me down.

I told them the basic history of my illness and my excitement of going to run the New York City Marathon for Team Fox. I also showed them the Team Fox promotional video that, not only talked about Team Fox, but showed clips of previous NYC Marathons. It was at about this point that I saw a cup being passed around their table and they started to put money into the cup and presented it to me to support Team Fox. I had found a new source of support and promised to come back and tell them how the marathon went.

Video Presentation at First Presbyterian Church

When I finally had Kristen's video and put it together with the video I had done, I wondered what it would be like. The day I finished putting it together, Julie and I had a small group meeting with friends from our church and I thought I'd ask them if they would preview it. They were very aware of our running the NYC Marathon for Team Fox.

When they saw the first few scenes, their first thoughts were surprise at the technological skills I had to put this together. After about five minutes of viewing, one of the ladies asked if we could pause the video while she went and got a box of tissues. When they finished, their overall reaction was amazement and they felt it needed to be shared with others.

The following week I had arranged to meet with First Presbyterian Church to talk about our marathon experience. We met during the Sunday school hour between the two services. Many of these were folks who had supported us financially as well as prayerfully.

The week leading up to the marathon, so many people told me or sent me notes saying that they were going to be praying for me at the exact time on Sunday in which we would be running. It got me to thinking, "Is there really any power in these prayers? Can it really have a physical effect, or is it intended to be the Christian way of wishing you well?" All I know is that at the 13 mile mark in the marathon, things were really starting to get bad, and every runner knows that it gets worse in the second half. My pace had really slowed down. I told Kristen that this was getting embarrassing. For some reason I thought about those who said they'd be praying for me. I chuckled and thought, "How are those prayers going to help me now?" So I grabbed a sport drink and plowed forward. As we approached the Queensboro Bridge at mile 14, Kristen asked, "Dad, do you realize how much your pace has picked up? I don't know how you're doing it, but keep it up for as long as you can." We finished the second half of the race three minutes faster than the first half. How could that happen?

After talking about the basic itinerary of events, I told them about the dvd we had put together. I told them I wanted to show it to them during this session. I was prepared this time as I had placed boxes of Kleenex at various locations. Many were used. When we finished, I told them I had made copies for them to take home and to show it to family and friends. Many wanted to pay for them but I just wanted to get my message out. Some asked if they could take a copy for a friend or family member who could benefit from viewing it. I decided to send a dvd to each person who had supported us, along with a thank you letter. I was beginning to feel that I had something here. Maybe I could put various presentations together with this video and touch people's lives.

Video Presentation at Knox County Parkinson's Support Group

The next week I returned to the Knox County Parkinson's Support group. I had been using my own projector and sound system that I had used with Mount Vernon FCA, so all I needed was a blank wall and it provided a more theater effect than watching it on a television. I really didn't know how these folks would react. After a brief introduction and explanation of our dvd, I said I'd let it do my talking.

When I was finished, there was an eerie silence in the room. One older man with overalls, flannel shirt and John Deere hat, got up and started pacing and fidgeting in the back of the room. I thought maybe he was exhibiting some of his Parkinson's symptoms. I thought I'd break the silence by saying, "Does anyone have a question or comment?"

The old man in the back of the room cleared his throat and spoke up. "I have something to say but I don't think I can say it without crying."

He bit his lip to no success as he and the rest of us were brought to tears. It was ok because we were all brothers and sisters in the same battle. He finally pulled himself together enough to say, "We come here each month and hear from doctors who tell us the latest things science is finding about this disease. We hear from pharmacists that tell us about the latest drugs that are being developed to delay the progression of the disease. We hear from physical therapists who tell us about exercises we should do to improve our ability to keep moving and nurses who tell us how to put them all together to try to be as normal as possible. They all mean well, but this is the first time we've heard from someone who's walking the journey with us. Someone who knows what it is like to go to bed each night knowing things will be the same or worse tomorrow. He tells us how to live with Parkinson's. To admit who we are and make the best out of our lives. We can control our attitude. I know that no one in this room will run a marathon, but after seeing what this man has done, I know I can change my attitude and do more with my life."

It was a pretty amazing experience. I don't think I'll ever be glad to have Parkinson's disease, but I know I would never have had that kind of an impact on someone's life without having to travel the journey I've been on.

The summer of 2010 was a time of major transition for our family. Julie and I had just retired and we made a decision to move to Cincinnati to be near our two daughters who lived there. This was a major move from friends we'd made in thirty-five years in Mount Vernon. These were people with whom we had raised families. It was difficult. It was going to be a cultural change. As I told people, we moved next door to one daughter, were one mile from the other and two miles from where I grew up. It was an amazing adventure and I found that my journey with Parkinson's was not over yet.

Finneytown Cross Country Team

Shortly after moving in and meeting our new neighbors, I found that a young man across the street was a cross country coach at Finneytown High School, our local school district, as well as a local youth pastor. After exchanging running experiences and telling him about running marathons, I asked him if he'd like to watch a dvd that my daughter and I had made. I gave him one to take home. A few days later he stopped me and asked me if I would be willing to talk to his cross country team. He said I'd have to keep it secular as one had to be careful speaking of faith in the public schools.

The gathering was at a pre-race dinner prepared by the parents and held in a fellowship hall at the coach's church. After having our spaghetti, I was introduced and I looked over my audience. Many were junior high runners but there were also many high school runners. Many parents stood in the back staying out of the way. There was the expected whispering going on as I began, but it was a Friday night and they didn't know who this guy was and what was he going to say.

As soon as the video started and the music began to play, the chatter stopped and they became engaged in the video. But more surprising was the fact that many parents were really involved with the film and my message. I told them that we were new to the neighborhood and that Saturday night I was going to set up a drive-in theater in my front yard. I was going to drop a sheet from my garage door and project the dvd on the sheet. I planned to use this to meet some of our new neighbors and maybe raise financial support for my second NYC Marathon. At least some would learn why they saw me running around the neighborhood. I invited them to bring their friends, knowing they would never come.

When I finished, many of the students came up and thanked me before they left for the evening's football game. Then I noticed many parents waiting to come up to speak to me, many wiping tears from their faces. They spoke of people they knew with Parkinson's or some other similar disease, how on target I was in my thoughts, and that my running the marathon was very inspirational.

As the people left I realized that there was one young man waiting at the side of the room. It was obvious that he wanted to come up last. When he finally came up, he said with a certain degree of difficulty that his father-in-law had Parkinson's disease pretty badly and was battling depression. He was just about giving up on life.

"Could I bring him to your drive-in tomorrow night?" he asked.

"Of course you can," I replied.

The next evening as Julie and I set up chairs, complementary brownies and bottled water, the young man drove up and transferred his father-in-law out of the van and placed him squarely onto his walker. I assisted him to a seat and after a brief explanation as to what this presentation was about, I showed the dvd. After it concluded, I talked at length with the old man with Parkinson's. I tried as best I could to raise his spirit and give him a more positive attitude. I assisted him back into his van and the young man handed me a check to support my cause. I put it in my pocket and helped Julie put everything back in the house.

Julie made the comment, "How do you think it went out there? You spent a lot of time with that older man."

I told her about the events of the past two days. I then reached into my pocket and pulled out the check I had been given. It was for $500. It was the biggest contribution I had ever received, and I'd only known him for two days.

College Hill Presbyterian Church

In the fall of 2010, I made an appointment to speak with the pastor (Drew Smith) of the new church we had been attending for a few weeks, College Hill Presbyterian Church. After a while, I introduced my Parkinson's situation, and my involvement with Team Fox. I shared my running of the 2009 New York City Marathon and my plans to run it again in a few weeks. He felt that I had quite a story and that I should share it with the congregation when I returned from my upcoming NYC Marathon.

When I gave my talk at College Hill Presbyterian Church in Cincinnati, I was very unsure what to expect. I had just recently finished the 2010 NYC Marathon and had only attended that church for a few months. I had my Mount Vernon First Presbyterian Church sermon down pretty well, but I needed to talk about the 2010 journey and how Mike Dubin (the man I had met briefly after the 2009 NYC Marathon) had showed up, five minutes before our bus left for the starting line, as an angel sent by God as an answer to my prayers. It made for a great story. But it got better.

As I sat with the pastor (Drew Smith) in front of the first service, nervous as could be, I realized that I didn't have a bulletin. I had worried about how long I would talk so I needed to know what else was on the program. I told Drew that I was going to the back of the sanctuary to get a bulletin. As I started to head towards the ushers in the back, there, sitting in the third pew with a smile from ear to ear was Mike Dubin. He had come, by himself, from Ann Arbor, Michigan, leaving at 4:00 am to support me one more time. I couldn't believe it.

My family had just entered the church and had seen me talking with a strange young man by the side aisle but I didn't let on. I guess Kristen said to Julie, "That man looks like the guy on dad's plaque hanging on his wall." When I got back to my seat, I leaned over to Drew and said, "Something has just happened that I have to share with the congregation. My sermon just became a little longer."

When I got done talking about how Mike Dubin had showed up unexpectedly on that bus in Manhattan that morning in November, I said to the congregation, "Something has happened unexpectedly this morning that I hadn't planned and I feel that I need to share it with you. It says in the book of Hebrews to always show hospitality to strangers, because many have entertained angels without knowing (Hebrews 13:2). I don't know if any of you have entertained an angel or not, but I'd like to introduce you to mine, who came down unexpectedly this morning from Ann Arbor, Michigan to support me one more time...Mr. Mike Dubin." As I went to give Mike a hug and thank him, all I remember is hearing someone in the congregation gasp, and then they rose as one and gave us a standing ovation. It was something I had never seen or experienced before or since. It made it difficult to conclude my sermon.

I concluded by stating what I had learned in my two years running for Team Fox. First, I repeated that I didn't look at my cup as half full or half empty, but that it was so full of blessings, things I never earned or deserved, filled with things people had done for me that I could never pay back, but maybe could pay forward. My cup was so full of blessings that they were overflowing and I needed to sip them out of the saucer.

I then told them, "Jesus Christ had a cup also. It was pure and without blemish. On the night that He was betrayed, He knelt in a garden and prayed. He prayed with such intensity that He sweat drops of blood...while His teammates slept in the bleachers.

And as He prayed, He looked into His cup. Do you know what He saw? He saw a crown of thorns. He saw Himself being beaten and spit upon. He saw the nails in His hands and feet. He saw the cross and the crucifixion. But you know what else He saw? He saw the sins of Matt Wilbur...all of them. He saw my sins and He saw your sins.

And being divine but totally human, He reacted like we might react. Twice He shouted at His father. 'Take this cup from me, I don't want it and I don't deserve it. But Thy will be done.'

And Jesus Christ paid it forward. He paid it forward 2000 years so that my cup and your cup could be pure and without blemish.

What was it He said just a few hours earlier to His teammates, at the pregame meal? Didn't He say something about being the cup of a new covenant offered to you? "Take my cup and you will do greater things than I ever did. Take my cup and you will never die but have everlasting life. Take my cup and I'll go and prepare a place for you in my father's kingdom, where there are no more tears, no more sickness and no more pain."

"Lord you have assigned me my portion and my cup; You have made my lot secure." *(Psalms 16:5)*

Miscellaneous Presentations

I spoke at several other venues to several types of groups. I spoke at a Cincinnati Tri-Wellness Parkinson's support group that I had been attending. Once again we were a band of brothers and sisters fighting in the same war on different fields of battle. We were walking the same walk. But once again, they seemed to be in a different place than I was. I didn't feel comfortable talking about the medications I took and the special accommodations I had to incorporate into my daily lifestyle in order to function. I showed them our video and they had the same emotional response. They received hope in seeing what someone in their situation had accomplished.

I also made a similar presentation at Llanfair Retirement Center where my father resided. I was speaking to that population that was cognitively capable of understanding my talk and video. Several significant things occurred which was particularly unique. While setting up for the presentation, an unrelated staff person just happened to be in the room as I tested the dvd for viewing and volume. I noticed that after a few minutes she had started to cry. I let the video roll and explained what it was about. She thought it would be so beneficial to these people. There was one lady who attended in one of those walkers that you turn around and sit on, who appeared particularly interested in the film and asked several questions afterwards. I was told later that I had had a real impact on her because she was usually a very bitter woman and felt cheated by her life's circumstances. One just never knows.

Chance encounters that lead to an opportunity to share my story have become the norm in my life. Many times people would visit our home to provide some service. They had come there to perform a job, but somehow the conversation would move to health, exercise, running or making the most out of our life, and I would introduce our dvd and offer them one to take home. I have had people see one of my NYC Marathon plaques and the conversation will turn to my story.

Cincinnati Christian Elementary School

Early in 2012, shortly after finishing the third (and what I had thought would be my final NYC Marathon), I started to feel a bit tired and sorry for myself. I didn't want to do these presentations any more. I didn't want to prepare another talk. I didn't want to be the "Positive Parkinson's Poster Boy for Team Fox". I didn't want to tell my story any more. Let someone else tell me a story. I didn't want to be someone's inspiration. Let them become their own inspiration.

Sure enough, that Sunday as I was feeling the joy of my new found freedom, a lady came up and asked if I could speak to the staff at the Cincinnati Christian Elementary School where she worked. She said it could only be about twenty minutes because it was a devotional time for teachers before school. I didn't have the courage to tell her I didn't want to do this anymore. And it would only be for twenty minutes. I could do that in my sleep. And I had made some shortened versions of our video and that would take a few minutes of the twenty minutes that I had, so I agreed to speak.

That morning I had to get up at about 6:00 am for a twenty minute drive across town, to a place I didn't really know the location of, and of course it was raining. I wasn't in a great mood. I told myself, "Do your thing, tell your story, show the video and get out of there. They have classes to go to so it can't run long."

A couple of minutes into my talk I heard the first sniffling. I told myself not to look up or make any eye contact. This would be over in a few minutes and I could go home. By the time the video was over the tears were hard to avoid. But it was over.

But they didn't leave. Didn't they have to go to classes?

One by one they came up and thanked me and told me of similar circumstances they were facing in their lives. One lady in particular was waiting in the back of the room trying to be last to come up. Finally, with tears running down her cheeks, she hugged me and told me how much my story meant to her.

"I've been carrying something in my heart that I haven't shared with anyone here. My husband is going to lose his job Friday and we don't know how we are going to face it. But your attitude and message has given me the hope to take home to my husband. Something wonderful is possible despite our present circumstances. I can't thank you enough. You are exactly what I needed today."

You think God was trying to tell me something? I guess I wasn't finished telling my story.

Wyoming Middle School

In 2012, I worked as a substitute teacher at Wyoming High School and Middle School. Subbing at the school I graduated from can be a little weird. It was particularly strange when I got called to sub at the middle school. I never taught at a middle school and to be honest, I never wanted to. Wyoming Middle School was where I went to high school. I had been the last high school class to graduate from that building.

My first day at the middle school was a surreal experience. I had to go in with all the demons I carried from that place. I walked past my old locker, my classrooms and the marble hall I had stood in before school my senior year. I didn't know how to get to the office, the restrooms or the teachers' lounge. I wasn't sure if I could find my classroom. By the time I got there, I wasn't sure if this was the middle school or the high school, whether it was 1971 or 2012. I was lost in space and time.

I couldn't wait until first period was over and I could splash some water on my face and figure out where I was. When the bell rang I headed towards the door in front of the kids. There standing in the doorway was a young woman I assumed was a teacher. "Don't tell me I am in the wrong room," I said.

"No. You're alright," she replied. "I just walked by and saw you and I wanted to know if you are Kristen Martin's dad."

What was going on here? I had just entered a strange place and someone is asking me if I was Kristen Martin's dad. "Yes, I am. How do you know me?"

"I heard you speak at our church in College Hill," she said. "I have your dvd and watch it quite often. I have a special needs child and it helps me maintain a positive attitude. I wanted to ask you if you ever speak outside of the church."

I said that I had quite often.

She asked that if she was able to set it up, would I be willing to speak to some of the seventh graders. She arranged with the health teacher for me to speak on a Monday. I wasn't sure they would really relate to my story. She assured me that they would and it might make them more sensitive to those with special needs. I suggested that from my experiences, adults have related to my story often and that she might want to invite any staff to come on their free period. She sent around a staff email suggesting that they give up their time grading papers and come and listen.

Giving these presentations meant I wasn't subbing but was in the classroom seven times in one day, and doing a presentation one time is emotionally tiring. I had started to like these middle school kids. They looked up to their teachers with respect and kindness. As I had hoped, each period consisted of about 25 little creatures and also about six or seven teachers, secretaries, administrators, custodians and other staff. I showed an adapted version of the dvd and told of my three years of marathons with Team Fox. I know I am getting old when the students don't know Michael J. Fox. As expected, as I showed my video many of the adults could be seen wiping their eyes. They could relate more to the problems all of us face in life. When finished, many of the adults thanked me and told of how they had a family member with Parkinson's or something similar and could really relate to what I had said. One young teacher said that he and his wife had been struggling and that he needed to hear a message from God that day and that he had just gotten the answer he needed.

I learned something that day also. The main message I tried to leave with the students was that we can't go through this life on our own. We are not strong enough. We are not smart enough. We need to depend on a strength or power stronger than us. We have to maintain a positive attitude at all times. And we have to leave ourselves open to the possibility that something wonderful could happen, despite the circumstances we find ourselves in. I suggested that walking through our life like that is exciting because as we walk down that hallway, we walk in anticipation that at any moment, around any corner, something wonderful could happen.

I realized that if we close a window, we prohibit the possibility of something wonderful happening. I realized that I had closed the window of running a fourth NYC Marathon and the wonderful things that may lie ahead. So I decided to run it again. I reminded myself that if running the NYC Marathon for Team Fox could touch the heart and spirit of other human beings, move them to a better place to be in their life, to give them a more positive attitude and help them become more of what God had created them to be, then I should keep running.

Eulogy For Irvin M. Wilbur - (my dad)

I had one more speech to give on May 4, 2012. It was the eulogy at my dad's memorial service. I have entered a copy of my speech. As always, I hope he was proud of his oldest son.

For those that don't know me, I'm Matt Wilbur and I am the oldest brother. I would like to say a few things about my dad. I will be speaking from my own perspective so I hope that most of what I say is the way my brothers saw things also.

My dad was a "Gentle Man", who always considered himself less than others and always cared for their needs before his own. He loved working in this church in many capacities from positions of leadership to working in soup kitchens to bringing shut-ins to church.

My dad laid a foundation for our lives by raising us up in "The Church"….this church. Boy Scouts, God and County, Sunday school and youth group activities were all a way of life growing up.

I grew up in an environment in which I never saw my dad smoke, drink, cuss or speak badly about anyone. As a youth, I may have seen that as a sign of weakness. When you grow up in a house with three boys, dinner time sometimes becomes a competitive event. If there was ever an extra hamburger or piece of chicken, it always went to one of the boys…never to dad…NEVER!

As each of the boys developed their unique interests, whether dad knew anything about them or not, he always made sure we had the opportunity to pursue our dreams. Whether it was equipping a dark room in the basement to develop photographs or providing piano lessons and a summer at Interlochen, he always provided us the opportunity to develop our talents. Dad had very few athletic skills. He probably didn't know if a basketball was "pumped or stuffed". But somehow a backboard got placed between two trees beside our driveway so a little boy could dream of being Bill Russell of the Boston Celtics going up against Wilt Chamberlin and the Philadelphia 76ers. Like every boy, I'd count down the last 5 seconds, take the last shot and if I missed…I was fouled.

One of the neat things about living where we do in Finneytown is that I can occasionally go out for a run over to 321 Fleming Rd. and check out the old homestead. I think it was about a year or so ago I ran past the house and they had cut down the trees that had held up my basket. All that was left was a pile of bark that they were probably going to use as mulch. I snuck up the driveway and took a few pieces of bark as a remembrance of a place that was so influential in my ultimate life choice. This is one of those pieces.

When I think about my dad's life, I always felt he deserved better. Living with my mom was, to say it kindly, difficult. She was ill much of the time and he had to be the caregiver even after his stroke and being in a wheelchair. He deserved better.

I'm sure that my brothers and I made parenting a nightmare. He deserved better.

And in his later years he went from being someone who had earned a good living, lived in a nice condo and made a good life for his family, to having a stroke, and living out the rest of his life in a nursing home without two nickels to rub together unless he won them at bingo. He deserved better.

But I came to learn that that is not the way Dad looked at his life. He loved and was devoted to my mom. She was the one with whom he created this family. His sons were a source of pride, whether it was hanging some of Paul's photographs on his walls, attending one of Allen's concerts or musicals or watching me shout out instructions from the sideline of a sport he knew very little about. It didn't matter if we won or lost, that was his son out there. He also enjoyed using his computer to track my progress in November as I ran 26.2 miles through the streets of New York City.

Although being in a nursing facility is something I wouldn't wish on anyone, he loved those who helped him and he always tried to make the most out of a tough situation. He always had a great attitude. I'd like to just take a moment to thank those that worked at Country Club Retirement Center in Mount Vernon and Llanfair Retirement Campus in College Hill for all they did for my dad. Those folks are a lot closer to heaven than I am.

Through my dad I learned that bad things happen to everyone. Many times it isn't our fault and we don't deserve it. We feel that we deserve better. But you know what, many times our lives are blessed and we did nothing to earn or deserve them either. Happiness comes when you decide to concentrate on the blessings and accept the grace that is given to you despite the fact that you don't deserve them.

I have been told that I have a disability (Parkinson's disease). But Dad's example has shown me that I am not disabled... "I'm more able." .... I am now "more able" to show compassion to those who have to overcome obstacles. .... I am "more able" to touch the heart and spirit of other human beings than I ever would have if I hadn't had my own trials to overcome.

If there is any good that I've done in my life, any joy or inspiration that I've given another human being, it's because of my dad.

Wednesday morning Julie and I were out running and somehow we ended up over at my old house. I noticed a new small tree had been planted where the older ones had been. It got me thinking. When I look at this piece of bark I ask the question, "Why did those trees have to be cut down?" Maybe they had some dead branches that kept falling on the ground or maybe it was too much trouble to rake up all those leaves. But didn't those old trees still have something to offer... even if it was just some cool shade during the hot Cincinnati summers. Maybe this is just the nature of life...that trees get old...are cut down...and soon replaced by a younger tree. All I know is that new tree is not strong enough to support a backboard...or the dreams of a little boy hitting a game winning shot for the Celtics at the buzzer.

Dad had similar questions, "Why have my limbs lost their strength? Why can't the doctors fix them?" I had no answers for him. He deserved better.

If I have any joy this morning, it's because I am assured of the fact that Dad's now in a place where he can get all the answers and living the life he's always deserved. .....Amen

Leave Yourself Open to the Possibility That Something Wonderful Can Happen

After the 2011 NYC Marathon, I had decided to call it quits in terms of running marathons. But one thing I had learned over the years was to leave ourselves open to the possibility that God may provide a beautiful opportunity for us despite our present circumstance. When I had an opportunity to speak to a group of 7th graders in 2012, I realized that maybe I was closing a window of opportunity for something wonderful to happen by deciding not to run the 2012 NYC Marathon. I saw that my story continues to touch lives. I decided to run the 2012 NYC Marathon. I have a strong feeling that this will be my last. I have no idea what God has in store for me. Kristen had said she would run it with me but she will be preparing to present us with another grandchild in December. Mike Dubin will be on a new journey, as he has decided to climb Mount Kilimanjaro for Team Fox. I thought that maybe I was meant to run this last one by myself, but I stayed open to the possibility that something wonderful could happen, despite my circumstances.

Joyce Chu is a doctor from Rochester, NY, whom I had met at earlier NYC Marathons. She ran for Team Fox as one of the five runners with Parkinson's disease. Although she is faster than me, she has contacted me and asked if I would like to run with her in the 2012 NYC Marathon. It might be neat to see two athletes with Parkinson's cross the finish line together. I will consider it a blessing to have such wonderful company helping me get to the finish line.

We're all on a journey to the finish line and we all need the help of family and friends to run the good race. Enjoy the journey.

Matt Wilbur's Words of Wisdom

1)	Everyone has a story to tell and if it's honest, humble and uplifting, people will want to listen. Sharing stories helps us connect with other human beings and acknowledge our shared feelings.

2)	Bad things happen to everyone, no one is exempt. Maybe "bad" is not the proper word but there are things that come into our lives that rob us of part of who we are. It might take some of our health, it might take some of our relationships or it might take some of our financial resources. The one thing it can't take from us is our attitude. That's ours to keep. And the great thing is that we get to make it anything we want it to be.

3)	When looking at the "cup" we've been given, some say, "Look what's been taken from my cup. It's half empty. There is hardly anything left in it. You can't expect me to accomplish or contribute anything with what's in my cup." And they usually don't. Another group says, "Yeh, something's been taken from my cup, but it's still half full, and there is still a lot there in which I can accomplish and contribute."

4)	My cup is not half empty or half full. My cup is so full of blessings, things I never earned or deserved…good things people have done for me that I can never pay back, but maybe can pay it forward. My cup is so full of blessings that they are overflowing and I have to sip them out of a saucer.

5)	When "bad" things happen, I look at my cup I say "How can I complain…the cup doesn't belong to me. It's been lent to me for 60, 70, maybe 80 years. Some things have been taken from my cup. There's some bad stuff in my cup. But there is some good stuff in there also. And it's my job to make the most out of what's in my cup, and give glory to God, who lent me the cup in the first place."

6)	Jesus Christ had a cup also. It was pure and without blemish. On the night that He was betrayed, He knelt in a garden and prayed. He prayed with such intensity that He sweat drops of blood, while His teammates slept in the bleachers.

And as He prayed, He looked into His cup. Do you know what He saw? He saw a crown of thorns. He saw Himself being beaten and spit upon. He saw the nails in His hands and feet. He saw the cross and the crucifixion. But you know what else He saw? He saw the sins of Matt Wilbur…all of them. He saw my sins and He saw your sins.

And being divine but totally human, He reacted like we might react. Twice He shouted at His father, "Take this cup from me, I don't want it and I don't deserve it. But Thy will be done."

And Jesus Christ paid it forward. He paid it forward 2000 years so that my cup and your cup could be pure and without blemish.

What was it He said just a few hours earlier at the pregame meal? Didn't He say something about being the cup of a new covenant offered for you? "Take my cup and you will do greater things than I ever did. Take my cup and you will never die but have everlasting life. Take my cup and I'll go and prepare a place for you in my Father's kingdom, where there are no more tears, no more sickness and no more pain."

7)   Walk through each of our days in such a way that we realize that we are not smart enough, strong enough or capable enough to get through this journey on our own. We need to find something or someone that we can depend on to help us on our journey. For me that is God, as I perceive Him. Keep a positive attitude and believe in the "possibility" that wonderful things can happen to us despite our present circumstances. When we live like this, life is exciting because we walk in the anticipation that at any moment, around any corner, there might be something wonderful ready to enter our life journey.

8)   I am only one, but I am one. I can't do everything, but I can do something. That which I can do, I ought to do. And that which I ought to do, by the grace of God, I will do.

9)   "Lord you have assigned me my portion and my cup;   You have made my lot secure." *(Psalms 16:5)*

ABOUT THE AUTHOR

Matt Wilbur grew up in Wyoming, Ohio. He received a BS degree from Miami University in 1975 with a major in math education and a minor in physical education. He also received a MEd from Ashland College in Sports Science in 1983. He was a high school math teacher and coach for 35 years while raising a family in Mount Vernon, Ohio.

Upon retiring in 2010, he and his wife Julie moved to Cincinnati, Ohio to reside near their two daughters: Kristen Martin and Cory Wilbur.

Matt can be contacted at mwilbur52@hotmail.com.